Mental Imagery in Health Care

Mental Imagery in Health Care

AN INTRODUCTION TO
THERAPEUTIC PRACTICE

Helen Graham
Lecturer in Psychology, Keele University, Staffordshire, UK.

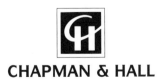

CHAPMAN & HALL

London · Glasgow · Weinheim · New York · Tokyo · Melbourne · Madras

Published by Chapman & Hall, 2–6 Boundary Row, London SE1 8HN, UK

Chapman & Hall, 2–6 Boundary Row, London SE1 8HN, UK

Blackie Academic & Professional, Wester Cleddens Road, Bishopbriggs, Glasgow G64 2NZ, UK

Chapman & Hall GmbH, Pappelallee 3, 69469 Weinheim, Germany

Chapman & Hall USA, One Penn Plaza, 41st Floor, New York NY 10119, USA

Chapman & Hall Japan, ITP-Japan, Kyowa Building, 3F, 2-2-1 Hirakawacho, Chiyoda-ku, Tokyo 102, Japan

Chapman & Hall Australia, Thomas Nelson Australia, 102 Dodds Street, South Melbourne, Victoria 3205, Australia

Chapman & Hall India, R. Sesadri, 32 Second Main Road, CIT East, Madras 600 035, India.

Distributed in the USA and Canada by Singular Publishing Group Inc., 4284 41st Street, San Diego, California 92105

First edition 1995

© 1995 Helen Graham

Typeset in 10/12 Times by Saxon Graphics Ltd, Derby
Printed in Great Britain by Page Bros (Norwich) Ltd

ISBN 0 412 56940 X   1 56593 333 8 (USA)

A Catalogue record for this book is available from the British Library

∞ Printed on permanent acid-free text paper, manufactured in accordance with ANSI/NISO Z39.48-1992 and ANSI/NISO Z39.48-1984 (Permanence of Paper).

Contents

Ancient origins of imaginative medicine

Logic can take you from A to B, but imagination encircles the world.
Albert Einstein

The sixteenth century French writer Montaigne commences his essay *Of the Power of Imagination* with the statement that a 'powerful imagination begets the thing itself', and supports this claim with numerous observations, both historical and personal. Citing the case of Gallus Vibius who 'so effectually bent his mind on understanding and imagining the nature and motions of madness that his judgement was thrown off its balance so that he never after recovered it' (Trechmann, 1927, p. 91), and noting that some commentators had attributed physical effects such as the scars of King Dagobert and the stigmata of St. Francis to imagination, he concluded 'it is likely that miracles, visions, enchantments and the like extraordinary phenomena derive their credit chiefly from the power of imagination'.

It was his contention, however, that not withstanding such exceptional incidents, the imagination is ordinarily quite powerful, and that everyone is struck by its 'strong arm', and some knocked down by it.

> We sweat, we tremble, we turn pale and blush through the shock of our imagination, and lying back in our feather-bed we feel our body agitated by its power, sometimes to the point of expiring. (Trechmann, 1927, pp. 91–2).

He confessed to being profoundly influenced by his imagination, and contriving to avoid it.

> I would live surrounded only by healthy and cheerful people. The sign of another's anguish gives me physical anguish, and my sensations often usurp those of a third person...I catch the malady which gives me concern and it takes root in me. I do not wonder that imagination brings on fevers and death in those who give it a free hand and encourage it. (Trechmann, 1927, p. 91).

He was in no doubt as to the potentially deadly consequences of a person's worst imaginings, relating the incident of a woman, who on being told in jest that she had eaten a cat pasty, 'was taken with a looseness of the bowels, accompanied by fever, and it was found impossible to save her' (Trechmann, 1927, p. 99). He also indicated that 'there are some who through terror, anticipate the hand of the hangman; and one whose eyes were being unbandaged to have his pardon read to him, was found stark dead on the scaffold, killed by the mere stroke of his imagination'. He considered that imagination killed passion as effectively as people, citing numerous incidences of male impotence which he attributed to this cause. Nevertheless, he recognized the imagination's power to cure as well as kill, and detailed ways in which it could be successfully employed to remedy this and other conditions.

A woman, imagining that she had swallowed a pin with her bread, shouted and raved as if she had an intolerable pain in her throat, where she thought she felt it sticking; an ingenious fellow, perceiving neither swelling nor any external alteration, and judging that it was all fancy and imagination, caused by a crumb pricking her in its passage, made her sick, and unseen, threw a bent pin into her vomit. The woman, thinking she had thrown up the pin, immediately felt herself eased of her pain. (Trechmann, 1927, p. 99).

Furthermore, Montaigne realized that physicians routinely employed powerful imagery when dealing with patients.

Why do the physicians begin by playing on the credulity of their patients with so many promises of cure, if not to the end that the power of imagination may assist the imposture of their decoctions? (Trechmann, 1927, p. 98).

He cited as a case in point that of a man normally prescribed several enemas who responded as effectively when the usual procedures were followed without administration of an enema. Montaigne therefore anticipated modern understanding of the role of the imagination in health, illness and healing, and the placebo effect, by some 400 years.

PHYSIOLOGICAL EFFECTS OF IMAGERY

It is only relatively recently that the physiological effects of intense imagery have been determined. During the 1920s the Russian psychologist Luria indicated that the mnemonist Shereshevskii could increase his heart rate by imagining himself running, and alter the size of his pupils and his cochlear reflex by imagining sights and sounds (Hunter, 1986). However, Jacobsen (1929) was the first investigator to establish that subtle tensions of small muscles or sense organs accompany imagery, and that appropriate motor neurons are activated when particular body movements are imagined. Shaw (1946) subsequently demonstrated that muscle tension increases in subjects who imagine lifting progressively heavy weights.

Later studies indicated that imagining eating a lemon has a direct effect on the production of the salivary glands (Barber, Chauncey and Winer, 1964), and that imagery can also elicit changes in blood sugar levels, gastrointestinal activity and blister formation (Barber, 1978). It was established that intense sexual and phobic imagery is accompanied by dramatic physiological changes (Laws and Rubin, 1969; Marks et al., 1971; Marks and Huson, 1973; Kazdin and Wilcoxin, 1975; Marzillier, Carroll and Newland, 1979; Stock and Geer, 1982; Smith and Over, 1987); that changes in heart rate, galvanic skin response, respiration and eye movement are associated with negative images; and that images of sadness, happiness, anger and fear can be differentiated by cardiovascular changes (Schwartz, 1973; Schwartz, Weinberger and Singer, 1981). Research (Schneider et al., 1988) also suggested that aspects of immune functioning could be influenced by imagery.

More recently the effects of imagery on various physiological functions, notably heart rate, blood pressure, blood flow, electrodermal activity and immune response have been confirmed. Many studies have reported an increase in heart rate in response to images of emotional and/or physical arousal (Craig, 1968; Schwartz, 1971; Waters and MacDonald, 1973; Gottschalk, 1974; Bell and Schwartz, 1975; Blizard, Cowings and Miller, 1975; Jones and Johnson, 1978, 1980; Bauer and Craighead, 1979; Jordan and Lenington, 1979; Shea, 1985); and decreased heart rate in response to relaxing imagery (Bell and Schwartz, 1975; Furedy and Klajner, 1978; McCanne and Iennarella, 1980; Arabian, 1982; Shea, 1985).

Increases in electrodermal activity have also been demonstrated in response to images of emotional and physical arousal (Stern and Lewis, 1968; Marks et al., 1971; Waters and McDonald, 1973; Gottschalk, 1974; Yaremko and Butler, 1975; Haney and Euse, 1976; Drummond, White and Ashton, 1978; Bauer and Craighead, 1979; Jordan and Lenington, 1979; Passchier and Helm-Hylkema, 1981); and experimental studies have confirmed that the diastolic blood pressure of normal subjects is raised in response to images of anger; and systolic blood pressure elevated by images of both anger and fear (Schwartz, Weinberger and Singer, 1981; Roberts and Weerts, 1982).

Experimental studies have also demonstrated changes in blood flow in association with imagery (Dugan and Sheridan, 1976; Kunzendorf, 1981, 1984; Okhuma, 1985), while clinical studies have shown that vivid images can be used to either increase internal blood flow or decrease external bleeding (Lucas, 1965; Willard, 1977; Chaves, 1980).

Within the past 10 years, experimental and clinical studies have confirmed earlier suggestions that immune functioning may be influenced by imagery. Siegel (1986) reports that the response of white blood cells and the efficiency of hormone responses to standard tests of physiological stress can be enhanced by appropriate imagery; increasing the number of white blood cells in circulation and the levels of thymosin-alpha 1, a hormone especially important to the T-helper cells. Other indices of improved immune function have also been reported in response to imagery (Hall, Longo and Dixon, 1981; Rider, Floyd and Kirkpatrick, 1985; Smith *et al.*, 1985; Schneider *et al.*, 1988); and an editorial in *The Lancet* (Anonymous, 1987) notes that patients recovering from cancer and AIDS owe much to the effects of imagery on immune function.

These findings prompted an awareness that it might be possible to control physiological functions, formerly thought to be autonomic or involuntary, by imagery, and to harness this ability more systematically in the treatment of illness. As Taylor (1987, p. 36) observes:

> If your teeth can be set on edge at the thought of a fingernail scraped on a blackboard, or your mouth can water at the thought of a Marmite sandwich, if you can become sexually aroused by erotic fantasies, that mental power can be harnessed. And if you accept...that the mind plays a very creative part in the formation of disease, so it follows that the mind can play an equally creative part in its eradication.

Indeed, studies have demonstrated that heart rate can be controlled, blood pressure lowered and homoeostatic balance achieved by way of imagery (Grossberg and Wilson, 1968; Revland and Hirschman, 1976; Carroll, Baker and Preston, 1979; Carroll, Marzillier and Merian, 1982; Engel, 1979; Lang *et al.*, 1980; Achterberg, 1985). In applied research, Burish and Lyles (1981) successfully used relaxing imagery to reduce systolic blood pressure in patients receiving chemotherapy for cancer. Ahsen (1978) and Crowther (1983) have also reported inducing long-lasting reductions in the systolic and diastolic blood pressure of hypertensive patients using relaxing images. Imagery has also been shown to increase the likelihood of cancer remission and regression (Fiore, 1974; Achterberg, Simonton and Simonton, 1977; Simonton, Matthews-Simonton and Creighton, 1978; Simonton, Matthews-Simonton and Sparks, 1980; Achterberg and Lawlis, 1979; Meares, 1981; Achterberg, 1984; Hall, 1984; Pickett, 1987-1988); to relieve pain, nausea and anxiety in cancer patients (Bradley and McCanne, 1981; Oldham, 1989); and reduce the side effects of cancer chemotherapy (Donovan, 1980; Lyles *et al.*, 1982). Furthermore the therapeutic uses of imagery have been applied in a variety of health care settings and validated on patients suffering from a wide range of physical and psychological illnesses (Achterberg and Lawlis, 1978; Sheikh, 1984; Achterberg, 1985; Siegel, 1986, 1990).

Dossey (1982, p. 67) therefore claims that the effects associated with imagery are 'as real as those produced by any drug', and that the processes of the imagination are potent therapeutic agents, or 'medicine' in the truest sense of the word. This understanding is precisely that on which traditional medicine throughout the world has been based since the earliest times, and which led Achterberg (1985) to describe shamanism (the oldest and most widely practised system of healing in the world) as the medicine of the imagination.

SHAMANISM – THE MEDICINE OF THE IMAGINATION

In most archaic traditions of the world one encounters the idea of some animating principle or force, a soul or spirit. This gives shape and structure to human life, influencing, directing and regulating it, while functioning below conscious awareness. The processes of this force are to a great extent unknown to the conscious mind but communicate with it by way of feelings, intuitions, dreams and imagery. Throughout history this inner world has been commented on by poets and philosophers. It has long been the province of religion, and occultism, which is concerned with the development of techniques for accessing this hidden realm and applying the knowledge acquired thereby. Mastery of methods for divining the inner world is traditionally the aim and purpose of shamanism, whose priests or shamans claim to be able to enter into this 'underworld'. There they commune with energies they characterize in various ways as human or animal spirits. These spirits are cultivated as 'inner guides' to help the shamans explore the inner world of others. Numerous means are used, all of which essentially put the shamans beyond ordinary conscious processes, and thus out of their minds in the normal sense, and in contact with what might be thought of as living energies containing information and ideas. The application of which in the mundane world constitutes the science or knowledge on which the practices of shamanic healing or medicine are based.

Shamanism in the strict sense is pre-eminently a religious phenomenon of Siberia and Central Asia, although it is not confined to those regions. The term derives from *shaman* which was introduced to the West in the seventeenth century by Russians who first encountered the Tungus of Siberia. The magico-spiritual life of these tribes centred on an individual known as the saman or haman, to whom various powers were attributed, including mastery of natural lore, healing the sick, telepathy, clairvoyance, divination of the future, dream interpretation, mastery of fire, rain making and communication with spirits. This person was not simply a practitioner of magic and medicine believed to cure and perform miracles, but also a priest, mystic and poet. In many tribes the shaman co-existed alongside other priests and magicians but nevertheless remained the dominating figure by virtue of the fact that he or she alone was the master of ecstasy, a trance-like or out-of-the body state, during which the soul was believed to leave the body and ascend to the sky or descend to the underworld in order to help members of the community in various different ways.

'For instance, the shaman may journey for the purpose of diagnosing or treating illnesses; for divination or prophecy; for acquisition of power through interaction with spirits, power animals, guardians or other spiritual entities; for establishing guides or teachers in non-ordinary reality, from whom the shaman may solicit advice on tribal or individual problems; or for contact with the spirits of the dead' (Harner, 1988, pp. 7–8).

This ability to journey in non-ordinary reality (to enter at will into an altered state of consciousness or expanded awareness) is the defining characteristic of the shaman which distinguishes him or her from other magicians and medicine people of primitive societies (Eliade, 1989). Whereas priests and medicine people work basically in ordinary reality, the shaman 'journeys and works in another reality while in a substantially altered state of consciousness' (Harner, 1988, p. 9). By so doing the shaman plays an essential role in the community, combating not only disease but demons and the power of evil.

> In a general way, it can be said that shamanism defends life, health, fertility, and the world of 'light', against death, diseases, sterility, disaster, and the world of 'darkness' (Eliade, 1989, pp. 508–9).

Thus, as Epes-Brown (1985, p. 397) observes, the shaman's powers are critical to communal life and human survival, helping people to maintain the necessary delicate balance 'between the world of pragmatic necessities and the more subtle world of spirits; acting as an intermediary between these worlds', and thus maintaining psychic and ecological equilibrium.

Similar magico-religious phenomena to those first described and documented in the various countries of Central and North Asia, were later observed in North America, Polynesia and elsewhere, and are still to be found throughout the world. Among the best documented by anthropologists are those of Australian Aborigines, who until the late eighteenth century, when Australia was colonized by West Europeans, had been almost totally isolated from the rest of humanity for tens of thousands of years, and were still living in a Stone Age culture. Contemporary descriptions of such practices in Polynesia (Freedom Long, 1954; King, 1983), Tibet (Eliade, 1989), India (Kakar, 1984); Australasia and Indonesia (Watson, 1976), North America and the Arctic (Eliade, 1964; Bergman, 1973; Epes-Brown, 1985), Central America (Castaneda, 1973, 1975, 1976, 1978, 1982, 1984); Africa and Australia (Taylor, 1987; Kalweit, 1988), Japan (Reid, 1985), China (Saso, 1985), Indonesia and Oceania (Eliade, 1989; Watson, 1976), together with archaeological evidence, confirm that shamanism is very ancient (many thousands of years old) widespread and remarkably similar throughout the world.

On the basis of their analysis of shamanic practices in 42 cultures, Peters and Price Williams (1980) have concluded that shamanic ecstasy is a specific altered state of consciousness or trance. Achterberg (1985) identifies it with what LeShan (1982) terms 'clairvoyant reality', which he claims is experienced by both mystics and healers, and describes as a timeless reality, a unified whole, where neither time nor space can prevent information exchange. Watson (1973, p. 218) similarly observes that all shamans seem to be able to see through the filters of culture, language and sense systems to other aspects of the real world, to hidden non-ordinary reality. Australian aborigines call this using the strong eye. According to Eskimo tradition, shamans also have the ability to generate and control internal heat.

> Every real shaman has to feel an illumination in his body, in the inside of

his head or in his brain, something that gleams like fire, that gives him the power to see with closed eyes into the darkness, into the hidden things or the future, or into another man (Achterberg, 1985, p. 218).

Indeed the shaman's essential role in the community depends above all on the ability to 'see' what is invisible to others and to provide direct and reliable information from this hidden or occult domain, for it falls to him or her to guard and defend the 'soul' of the community, whose 'form' and destiny he or she alone can 'see' (Eliade, 1989, p. 8), albeit in the mind's eye.

The spiritual vision of the shaman

In primitive societies the soul was conceived as 'permeating on earth, in the air and on the water, in all the diverse forms assumed by persons and objects, one and the same essential reality; both one and multiple, both material and spiritual' (Lévy-Bruhl, 1928, p. 16). This all-pervading quality unified man and nature and the present with the eternal because it was believed that the core of each person, his real self, belonged to the spiritual sphere, coming from a pre-existing world of spirits, descending from spirit ancestors, and returning after death to its spirit home, or 'eternal dreamtime' as it is termed by the Aborigines. The spiritual and sacred were not divorced from the natural world and the material body, however, because the material world was itself impregnated with spiritual qualities. The 'dreaming' or spirit realm therefore permeated all time and space and endowed the world with life and meaning. Accordingly the shaman perceives the soul or essence of man as integral to an infinite and eternal universe in which no part is separate from any other, all phenomena being an expression of an underlying unity, and man as a replica of it. The essential nature of man is therefore to live in harmony with the universe, and the aim and purpose of human life is to preserve the soul and maintain its integrity, harmony and balance. Failure to do so is disastrous as it renders life pointless and meaningless, as is indicated in the Aboriginal proclamation: 'He who loses his dreamtime is lost'. The shaman therefore functions to defend the psychic integrity of the community by keeping man in touch with his soul, nurturing and protecting it, and restoring it to those individuals who have lost sight of, or contact with it.

The latter process is generally conceived as a quest in which the shaman journeys through what might be regarded as the landscapes of the unconscious mind in search of the lost soul, which when found is returned to its owner. The shaman therefore evokes powerful imagery in himself and others as a means of accessing, exploring and interpreting these ordinarily inaccessible regions. Consciousness is thus withdrawn from the everyday world and shifted towards the inner world of images. Various techniques which have the effect of transferring consciousness from the outer sensory world to the inner are used to induce this trance state, including sensory and sleep deprivation and fatigue, fasting and breath control. Hallucinatory and stimulant drugs, drum music, dancing, rhythmic movement, chanting, incantation and other rituals may also be used to intensify perception, intuition and imagination in preparation for what Drury (1991), in the manner of Native American Indians, terms the vision quest: a 'journey which is visually a fact-finding mission aimed at discovering the cause of sickness, injury, drought, famine and so on. It is essentially a 'a dream of knowledge'' (Drury, 1987, p. 23). The shaman is thus someone who can control the trance dimension and explore the realms of the cosmos which are accessed by this altered state of consciousness, awaking from it 'with conscious memory of the journey to the gods or ancestral spirits, and full knowledge of magical cures or healing procedures' (Drury, 1987, p. 17).

To the shaman dis-ease or imbalance is an indication of spiritual crisis resulting from loss of personal power rather than any physical cause. Initially the shaman attempts to establish how the dis-eased individual has lost power. Shamans recognize that imagery (the processes of the imagination) is the product of what modern man calls the 'unconscious mind', and often reveals and verifies inner conditions hidden to ordinary consciousness. Accordingly images, the products of imagination, are often indicative of the ways in which individuals perceive themselves and their world, and as such provide significant cues to their spiritual health or robustness and their susceptibility to emotional and physical illness. Disempowering thoughts, attitudes and feelings, such as anxiety, fear and depression, may be discerned in a person's worst and wild imaginings. Shamans therefore attend to a person's spontaneous imagery as revealed in patterns of speech and language, fantasy and dreams. They may also stimulate or guide imagination so as to elucidate these features, and gain insight into the individual's condition and appropriate treatment. The latter focuses on augmenting the patient's personal power rather than treating physical symptoms, and is little concerned with combating illness-producing agents, that are seen to constitute a threat to health only when a person's power is weakened.

Imagery is used to increase personal power in various ways. The shaman may instruct the patient in the use of deliberate imagination, whereby strong imagery is used to direct beliefs, thoughts, emotions and actions more positively. The shaman may work directly on both the psychological and the physical aspects of disease by suggesting powerful imagery to the patient. Indeed, as Achterberg (1985) indicates, for shamans with little or no direct knowledge of anatomy and physiology, images are as much a physiological reality as any other body function, capable of both producing symptoms of disease and curing them. Shamans are thus adepts of 'imaginative medicine', who evoke and interpret vivid imagery in both diagnosis and treatment, and induce in others altered states of consciousness conducive to self-healing.

Mysticism and medicine

As an elite with access to a region of the sacred inaccessible to others, and by way of their ecstatic visionary experience, shamans have exercised, and still exercise, a powerful influence on religious ideology, mythology and rituals worldwide, and on the practices of healing. Importantly, however, these ideas, myths, rites and practices are not their creation. Indeed all the features of shamanism occurred prior to, or at least parallel with it, and arose in the first instance as a product of the *general* religious experience rather than that of a class of privileged person (Eliade, 1989, p. 7).

There are indications in ancient mythology and in various teachings that have been passed down through history, such as the *Huang Ti Nei Ching* or *The Yellow Emperor's Treatise on Internal Medicine* (c. 770–467 BC), that early man was inherently attuned to nature, and that he instinctively and collectively understood and lived in accordance with its fundamental forces. This wisdom was not a function of intellect or reasoning but of intuition. According to Jaynes (1993) this feature of the primitive mind is evident in ancient Greek mythology. He observes that the characters of Homer's *Iliad* do not sit down and think out what to do, or act on the basis of conscious plans, reasons and motives but auto- matically in accordance with the promptings of 'gods': 'They have no conscious minds such as we say we have, and certainly no introspections' (p. 72), and therefore, he claims, it is impossible for modern man to understand them or the universe they inhabited.

Certainly it would appear that non-verbal intuitive awareness of the whole- ness of things and the relations between all phenomena is a feature of pre-liter- ate cultures. This awareness has largely been lost by mankind during the course of intellectual evolution, as the parts of the brain specialized for language and language-related functions evolved and eclipsed those parts of the brain more specialised for non-verbal, holistic, intuitive processes. Colegrave (1979) insists that this loss is irrecoverable, but others such as Blavatsky (1988), Besant (1899), Freedom Long (1954), Gurdjieff (1978), Ashe (1977), Drury (1978, 1987) and Butler (1982) argue that this wisdom, although fragmented and obscured, has never fully disappeared, having been passed down the ages in various traditions, many of them secret. It therefore 'runs like an underground river emerging now and then into the light of day, then disappearing again beneath the surface' (Butler, 1982, p. 11).

Certainly the ancient mythology and history of many cultures supports the latter proposition. These traditions assert that man's vision of the universe is blinkered by conventional reality, or certain learned ways of perceiving, which confine his awareness to what is immediately apparent. They maintain that a far greater hidden or occult reality exists beyond normal awareness and ordinary comprehension; an infinite, everchanging, expanding, indivisible and ultimately indescribable universe of harmonious relationships and interrelationships, of which man is part, and which can only be perceived by those so attuned. These individuals with insight into the true nature of the universe and its mysteries are variously referred to as seers, visionaries or mystics – a term derived from the Greek verb *muo* meaning to close or complete. Mystics are therefore persons with a complete picture of reality, or cosmic vision. Mysticism refers to an experience of, or belief in, a reality surpassing normal human understanding or experience, which is fundamental to life.

The philosopher Bertrand Russell (1959) has indicated that throughout history and all parts of the world, mysticism is characterized by certain beliefs: the concept of a timeless reality beyond and utterly different from the world of ordinary appearance, knowledge of which comes by way of revelation, sudden insight or intuition 'certain beyond the possibility of doubt'; and awareness of the unity and indivisibility of all things. Magic can be considered applied mysticism inasmuch that mystic vision, awareness and sensitivity enables the individual to penetrate and understand the secrets of the universe, together with human nature and destiny, and to work with universal forces accordingly to produce desired effects at will. It was therefore to mystics, magicians and shamans that others turned with their problems. Hence they tended to control access to knowledge, to determine what would be disclosed and to whom, and the means of dissemination. Given the ineffable quality of the vision of mystics, they often taught by analogy or metaphor, and used practices aimed at enhancing consciousness in others so that they might apprehend ultimate reality directly. The process was essentially that of developing insight or inner vision in order to benefit from intuition, or, quite literally, inner knowledge or teaching. These visionaries were therefore the first educators and their insights form the basis of human civilization as we know it.

Certainly mysticism informed the practice of medicine throughout the world, as is clearly discernible in the healing traditions of most cultures, especially those of the East where thinking remains close to its mystical origins.

THE TRADITIONS OF THE EAST

Indian philosophy and teaching

Vedanta, the philosophy expounded in the earliest scriptures of the Hindu (the Persian word for Indian) comprises all the various sects of India. It derives from the Vedas, ancient teachings or knowledge (from the Sanskrit *vid* which means to know) and is a practical philosophy rather than a mere intellectual understanding, in which reality must be directly known and this knowledge applied in daily life. Vedanta therefore teaches that life has no other purpose than learning to know ourselves for what we really are, a manifestation of the Ultimate Reality or Brahman. This one great, impersonal and absolute power is conceived as an immutable, ultimate and essentially indescribable reality which pervades and transcends all things, unifying all the apparent differences of the phenomenal world. It is the first principle from which all things derive, by which all are supported, and into which they eventually disappear. Indeed, all phenomenal existence is viewed as transitory, impermanent and in the process of change. Stutley (1985) indicates that a frequent metaphor for Brahman is 'ocean' which denotes inexhaustible potentiality. Like the ocean the greater part of Brahman is never visible or known, and like its rising and disappearing waves the ephemeral lives of the myriad creatures come into existence for a while and then are resorbed into it.

Vedanta teaches that by personal effort and use of inner knowledge man can attain union with Brahman while alive. This is possible because Brahman and the individual soul or atman, though seemingly apart, are in actuality one, as is conveyed in the teaching: 'The real is one. It is the mind which makes it appear as many'. This illusion, or maya, disappears when direct knowledge of Brahman is attained. Understanding maya, the illusory nature of reality, is therefore of key importance in Vedanta, the aim of which is to harmonize all.

Imagery has been employed to this end within Indian traditions for thousands of years. Vedanta recognizes that the human mind is incapable of conceiving the Ultimate Reality with which it seeks union and that it therefore turns to imagining either a God or gods with attributes which are the projections of human virtues, or exemplary individuals. These images are worshipped in the hope that through devotion the worshipper can become like them. A person may therefore imagine a certain god or object and repeatedly focus on it until it becomes vivid; a process which may take many years, after which he or she will attempt to identify with it. Vedanta does not condemn such practices but reminds worshippers that the god or exemplar must not come between them and the knowledge that they are all essential projections of the same Ultimate Reality, and that in worshipping those in whom eternal nature is revealed, they are revering their own divine nature which is more or less obscured. Fundamentally, therefore, 'Vedanta teaches men to have faith in themselves first' (Vivekenanda, 1974, p. 6), and this is reflected in traditional Indian medicine, Ayurveda.

Imagery in Ayurvedic medicine

The tradition of Ayurveda, which is claimed as the grandfather of all holistic health systems, is some 3000 years old. Until the formation of the British Empire, when Western medicine overtook India, it was dominant on the Indian sub-continent. Since India regained independence in 1945 there has been a remarkable resurgence of interest in this system.

Ayurveda, and its offshoot Unami which is dominant in Pakistan, have become known in the West only recently through its practice within immigrant Asian communities. In 1980 the World Health Organization suggested that its principles should be widely known as they could help to integrate complementary and orthodox Western medicine.

Ayurveda is Sanskrit for the 'science of life' and it is a section in the last four

Vedas, the Atharva Veda, written about 1200 BC. Although its early history is obscure it contains magical spells and charms to treat a wide range of natural and supernatural conditions, suggesting origins in early magic. Moreover, as Ancient India had no writing, all its teachings were memorized and handed down orally by the highest caste, the Brahmins, in characteristic occult tradition. The first school of medicine was established at Banares in 500 BC and the main texts *Susruta Samhita* and *Charaka Samhita* were written there in 5 and 6 BC, respectively. Together they constitute a comprehensive system of medicine which is essentially cosmological in considering health as a harmonious balance between constituent qualities and energies of man and the universe. Its fundamental premise is that man must be regarded as a whole, with no separation of mind, body and soul.

A central practice of Ayurveda is yoga, which is not, as some Westerners suppose, merely a system of physical exercise but a complete philosophy and self-help system which embraces the whole person in their physical, mental and spiritual aspects. The term itself derives from the Sanskrit *yuj*, meaning to join or yoke, and it signifies the union of the individual with the Ultimate Reality. It is therefore essentially a spiritual discipline; a means of attaining the highest aim of Vedanta and Hindu culture.

There are many different forms of yoga. Hatha yoga is concerned with integration through strength, whereby the body is brought to the peak of health and efficiency through physical and breathing exercises. Jnana is meditation on sacred texts. Bhakti is intense devotion to a chosen deity. Karma is integration through good works and action. Raja aims to control the subconscious mind. Other forms of yoga are Mantra, Kundalini, Laya and Tantra.

Mantra yoga is based on the inherent healing power of sound and vibration as revealed by ancient seers. It aims to alter ordinary consciousness by rhythmic repetition of divine names or phrases known as mantra, which may be used alone but are more generally combined with other techniques, including imagery. A mantra may therefore be repeated as a person imagines healing light (Clifford, 1984), or imagined as a mandala, a complex circular pattern which represents symbolically the intricacies of the Ultimate Reality and the principles with which the devotee strives to identify, and is considered to confer healing when held in the hand or in the heart (Sheikh, Kunzendorf and Sheikh, 1989).

The aim of Kundalini yoga is the arousal of cosmic energies enabling the individual to merge with Ultimate Reality. It involves the attainment of mastery of the senses and the generation of intense bodily heat. It achieves its aim primarily by way of meditation and imagery, and as such is clearly consistent with shamanic practices.

Tantra is also a refinement of shamanic practices and endeavours to overcome and thereby dominate the distractions of the world that stand between the individual and the absolute by using them to destroy the desire for sensual experience. Imaginative methods are commonly used, including meditation on mandalas.

Imagery in Tibetan Buddhism and medicine

Imaginative exercises which derive from ancient Tantric texts are also a feature of Buddhism, notably that of Tibet (Evans-Wentz, 1967). Typically these direct the person to imagine being 'eternally in the shape of a deity', the precise details of which are vividly and meticulously specified as in the manner of guided fantasy; or involve mandalas.

In the West, Buddhism is generally viewed as a characteristic Indian tradition, and while it is the case that it emerged from Hinduism as a dominant philosophy of the Indian sub-continent it is generally less influential in India than elsewhere. Wilson-Ross (1973) indicates that although in time Buddhism was resorbed into the all-embracing Hindu tradition from which it sprang it was destined to become and remain the dominant influence in vast regions of Asia, Sri Lanka, Burma, Cambodia, Thailand, Vietnam, Laos, Tibet, Mongolia, China, Korea and Japan, 'where it has had an almost incalculable effect on art, literature and ways of life'. Over 50% of the world's population live in areas where Buddhism has at some time been the dominant philosophical force. Moreover, Buddhism is an evolving tradition extending over two and a half millennia and no other philosophical tradition has existed in such disparate cultures as a major influence for so long.

Buddhism originated in about the sixth century BC in the teachings of the Indian sage Siddhartha Gautama, the Buddha or Awakened One, so called because he was regarded as one who had 'woken up' to the true nature of reality, and the basic truth of the universe. Buddha emphasized the importance of self-awareness or insight as the means by which man may realize his true nature as a manifestation of universal one-ness and attain harmony with it. In the Buddhist tradition insight is developed by way of various techniques. In what is known as the Theravada School of Buddhism there are two stages: satipatthana, in which the mind is trained to see things as they are, without emotion or thought; and satpatthana, in which the mind is brought under control by way of concentration and attention. Exercises in self-control may involve focus on external or internal features such as breathing, emotions and images. Only when self-control is achieved does the person progress to the third stage, known variously as vipassana, satori or samadhi; an utterly impersonal awareness of the object of observation such that 'the observer becomes the essence of the thing observed' (Humphreys, 1962). Only when the truths of the Theravada School have been assimilated can the individual grasp the expanded and deeper truths of the Mahayana School which has flourished in Tibet, Mongolia, The Himalayas, parts of China and the Soviet union, Japan and Korea.

Mahayana Buddhism forms the basis of Tibetan medicine, which reflects the belief that health is a state of balance between man and the universe.

Human illness, however minor, is seen as a cosmic event. As a body man is a microcosmic but faithful reflection of the macroscopic reality in which he is embedded and which preserves and nourishes him every second of his life; as a mind, he is a ripple on the surface of a great ocean of consciousness. Health is the proper relationship between the micro- cosm which is man and the macrocosm which is the universe. Disease is a disruption of this relationship. (Yetsehe Dhonden, personal physician to the Dalai Lama, cited in Anderson, 1982, p. 219).

The aim of Tibetan medicine is to restore harmony and balance. Healing is therefore essentially spiritual and the leading physicians are lamas or monks. Healing practices are complex and often elaborate, and diverse imaginative methods are employed in which mental images are formed or visualized. A widely used visualization exercise involves the mandala of the medicine Buddha.

At the centre of the mandala, a radiant Buddha sits in a lotus position on a 1000-petalled lotus, which in turn is perched on a jewelled throne. In his right hand he is holding the myrobalan plant, and in his left hand a begging bowl filled with healing nectar. In this exercise, one imagines that one is sitting in a beautiful landscape and offering to the Buddha all that is precious. Now one asks him for his blessing and to sit on the top of one's head. Then one senses the Buddha's rays of brilliant light stream into the body, dissolving illness and suffering (p. 480).

A variation is to visualize oneself as the medicine Buddha and the outer world as the outer part of the mandala. Thus one generates the healing light of the Buddha and thereby one's view of the self and the world is purified (Sheikh, Kunzendorf and Sheikh, 1989, p. 481).

The visualization of light plays a large part in Tibetan medicine. Brilliant white or coloured light is imagined radiating from a deity and flowing through one's being, purifying it both mentally and physically. The light can be directed by the person to a diseased area of his or her body, or outwards into the universe if healing others.

Another healing meditation involves Buddha Vajrasattva, a deity of purification. He is white, sitting in lotus position, holding in his right hand a vajra, representing skilful means, and in his left hand a bell, representing wisdom. One imagines him to be sitting on the top of one's head and confesses one's transgressions to him. Then by the strength of one's promise to avoid further wrongdoing and due to Vajrasaava's vow to purify, his light streams into one's head and descends into the body illu- minating it. All of one's mental and physical ailments dissipate and exit one's being in the form of blood, pus, smoke and insects (Sheikh, Kunzendorf and Sheikh, 1989, p. 481).

Imagery in Chinese medicine

Like the Hindus and the Tibetans the Chinese have always recognized a magic link between man and the world, viewing both as parts of a sacred metabolic system. In their view the cosmos is an organic unit which spontaneously evolved the manifest and unmanifest worlds. This cosmic source, or Tao, roughly translated in English as 'the Way'. Symbolized by white light, it is at once the primal principle of the universe and the way to achieve personal realization of it. It is the most ancient and fundamental concept in Chinese thought. Instructions as to the way of producing light within the self are therefore implicit in its two classic philosophies, Taoism and Confucianism which broadly represent the two sides of Chinese character, the mystical and practical respectively.

Taoism pre-dates Confucianism, and its sources are uncertain. However elements of pantheism and magic suggest origins in mysticism. The teachings of the way were formally expounded in the doctrines of Lao Tzu in about 600 BC and later expanded by Chuang Tsu. The *Tao Te Ching*, or *Book of Changes* attributed to them, centres on the concept of chi, ch'i or qi which refers to the vital energy which animates the Tao or cosmos. Man is seen as infused with the powers of the universe, as a microscopic image of the macrocosm, and like the cosmos as a whole, the body is seen as being in a state of continual, multiple and interdependent fluctuations the patterns of which are described in terms of the flow of chi. The *Tao Te Ching* therefore teaches that the task of the sage is to create a conscious harmony between himself and the cosmos, so that his or her chi resonates with that of the environment. This state of harmony and wholeness is synonymous with health; all illness being regarded as the result of imbalance in the flow of chi. Taoism therefore aims at maximizing the harmonious flow of chi in and around the person. However, because man is imbued with all the powers of the universe, wisdom is considered to reside within the person rather than externally, and is achieved primarily by insight, or looking inwards. Insight is therefore a precondition of wholeness or health. Traditional Chinese medicine therefore uses various techniques to promote the flow of chi and awareness of this process, including imagery.

Individuals are encouraged to enhance, redirect and normalize chi by imagining it in various ways. Chi is commonly conceived as the vital energy or breath which animates the cosmos. Hence considerable emphasis is placed on energizing the individual through correct breathing. In Chinese martial arts traditions, for example, a common breathing exercise is to imagine breath being drawn in through the nose as light and travelling down the spine to a point approximately two inches below the navel, referred to as T'ian, T'ein or the golden stone, before being drawn up through the chest and out of the mouth. The image of fog or nothingness filling the body from bottom to top may also accompany deep breathing. T'ai Chi Chuan, a system of exercises designed to promote the flow of chi through the body–mind, also incorporates specific images of chi. A feature of perhaps the best known technique of Chinese medicine, acupuncture, is that the practitioner imagines blending his or her chi with that of the patient during treatment.

Imagery in Japanese medicine

Japanese medicine corresponds very closely with that of China. The indigenous physicians of early Japan having been displaced by the Chinese by the ninth century AD. Acupuncture is widely practised, as is Shiatsu which uses firm physical pressure in treatment. A form of therapy becoming more widely known in the West is Reiki. This was developed during the last century and involves the channelling and balancing of universal life energy, or Ki as it is known in Japan, within oneself and from person to person, through the hands by way of visual images and symbols.

The relationship between Eastern traditions

Clear correspondence may be discerned among the philosophies of China, Japan, India and Tibet, and in the principles and practices of healing which derive from them, notably in their emphasis on the importance of insightful awareness and the use of imagery. Motoyama (1987) has concluded that despite differences in terminology the concepts on which the healing traditions are based and the fundamental reality with which they are concerned are the same. Certainly several common themes can be identified in the traditions of the East. They all emphasize the illusory nature of everyday reality and the inter-relatedness of everything. They also share an awareness of subtle energies within the universe, with which man is imbued, and they all aim at achieving balance of the forces within man, and between man and the environment. This integration or whole-ness is synonymous with health and holiness, and reflects the common belief that the physical, emotional and spiritual aspects of man are one; that there is no separation between body and mind, nor between the individual and the universe. All are intimately and dynamically related. Typically, therefore, Eastern tradi-tions are characterized as religious or philosophical. However, as Watts (1961, p. 19) observed, the psychological window is the best one from which to view the traditional wisdom of the East because 'if we look deeply into such ways of life, we do not find either philosophy or religion as these are understood in the West, we find something more nearly resembling psychotherapy'.

Certainly in all the traditions of the East the mind is considered intrinsic to disease of all kinds, and treatment is directed primarily to and through the mind, and only secondarily to the body. By contrast, in the West, where mind and body are generally regarded as two largely distinct realms it might be supposed that mental processes such as the imagination have little or no part in 'physical' matters of health and illness, and that medicine is a rational science based on understanding of physical processes. Nothing could be further from the truth.

IMAGERY IN EARLY WESTERN MEDICINE

Although the origins of Western medicine are shrouded in mythology the influence of mysticism, magic and shamanic practices are nonetheless discernible.

Ancient Egypt

Homer identified the Egyptians as more skilled in healing than any other people in the ancient world. Their medicine was rooted in the mystical vision of a harmoniously interrelated universe suffused with the divine. Man was viewed as a microcosm of the macrocosm and expected to reflect its order and harmony. This was achieved through a balancing of subtle cosmic forces conceived as an expression of God, symbolized as light, and earthly forces, symbolized by a rearing serpent. (A similar concept is also symbolized in the Hindu tradition as a serpent and in the Chinese tradition as a dragon.) The most important aim in life was for man to become 'enlightened' by opening himself to the light, channelling and distributing it, and merging it with earth energy. Insofar as man achieved this union he was the mediator of heaven and earth, and the aim of magic was to produce this connection, thereby 'bringing down the light', transferring and reflecting its power (Jacq, 1985). The secrets of this ancient wisdom were passed on only to the highest order of priests for sole use in the service of man and his spiritual development. Magic and religion were thus intrinsically linked with each other and with medicine, which was largely the province of temple priests. In addition to the priests, there were various kinds of healer, from bonesetters to those who could tap into and direct natural forces, but the most highly prized were those with the ability to evoke and interpret dreams in both diagnosis and treatment. Imhotep, born circa 3000 BC, who was the most renowned master of magic, divination, herbal lore, poetry and rainmaking, clearly displays the shamanic origins of Egyptian medicine. On his death he was elevated to the status of a demi-god and later to a full deity of medicine, being designated the son of Ptah, god of healing. In his name Egyptian traditions of healing were passed on and found their way into ancient Greece.

Ancient Greece

Until the sixth century BC the aim of the Greeks was physis, the attempt to perceive the essential nature of all things. It was synonymous with mysticism and its practical applications consistent with magic. All knowledge or *scientia* (from which the term science derives) concerned understanding the meaning and purpose of natural phenomena and living in accordance with natural law. The concept of harmony was therefore of central importance to the Greeks, as was the related concept of measure. This was viewed not as an overt feature of phenomena but a deeper hidden harmony which was deemed to lie in the ratio of its inner proportions to one another and the whole. To understand this ratio and thus have the measure of a thing was a form of insight into its essential nature and harmony. Maintaining this sense of measure, proportion or rationality was vital to man whose essence, soul or psyche became fragmented and thus irrational when its right proportions were lost. All human problems were therefore seen as psychopathology in the literal sense of soul-sickness, that is, as disharmony or dis-ease of the soul. Physical disorders were largely regarded as symptomatic of this fundamental disharmony and treatment was therefore directed to the cure of the soul, or psychotherapy, through restoration of its balance and harmony. The legacy of this idea is found in the terms health and healing which originate in the German *heilen*, meaning whole, which is closely related to the Old English words *hael* (whole), and *haelen* (heal), from which the English hale (as in the phrase hale and hearty) and the Welsh hoil derive. These terms are very similar to the German heilig and the Old English halig meaning holy. Etymologically speaking therefore, to be healthy is to be whole or holy, which clearly embraces both the spiritual and physical aspects of man, and not merely the latter.

Such a distinction would have been meaningless to the early Greeks who did not even have a word for matter, since they regarded all forms of existence as manifestations of the physis, endowed with life and spirituality. All phenomena were deemed to be comprised of gods and spirits, and the universe to be a kind of organism sustained by pneuma or cosmic breath, in much the same way that the human body is sustained by air. Until about the sixth century BC gods and spirits were central to all thinking about the universe, as is reflected in Greek mythology, and healing was a spiritual phenomenon associated with these deities.

Three gods were seen as principally responsible for healing. Apollo, healer to the gods, who with his arrows, the rays of the sun, brought not only healing but also pestilence and death. His sister Artemis, on the one hand helper to women in childbirth and on the other the goddess of death. Pallas was the patron of eyesight. However, in the Homeric tradition this healing trinity is compounded by the myth of Asclepios, the son of Apollo and King of Thessally, who with his wife Epione, the soother of pain, created a dynasty of healers. His heroic sons Macaon and Podilirius were military surgeons, Telesporos brought about completion of the healing process, and his daughters Hygiea and Panacea were respectively the dispenser of health and the friendly goddess of the sick. Panacea had knowledge of medicines to treat disease, and Hygiea advocated living in harmony with nature in order to avoid illness.

It is in the cult of Asclepios (known by the Romans as Aesculapius) that similarities with Egyptian medicine can most clearly be seen. Asclepios, like Imhotep, has uncertain origins. There appears to have been a mortal physician of that name revered as the founder of medicine, who, on death, became first a demi-god then a full deity. The followers of the latter, Asclepiads, or the sons of Asclepios, were temple priests, and like the Egyptian priests, they worshipped the symbol of the rising sun. Moreover, Asclepios was typically depicted bearing the caduceus, or rustic staff around which is curled a serpent, representing earth energy. This later became the emblem of the physicians of Kos where the Hippocratic school of medicine was founded, and eventually that of Western medicine. Like the Egyptians, Asclepiads used dreams in diagnosis and treatment. Indeed they perfected dream therapy as a diagnostic and therapeutic tool. In preparation for dream therapy the sick fasted in order to attain the spiritual clarity necessary for the receipt of divine messages. After this they went to the temple, there to await the gods. Diagnosis and treatment took place during the state of consciousness just prior to sleep, when what are now referred to as hynogogic images would occur, bringing insight and healing. Many cures were ascribed to this procedure

> ...the blind, lame, deaf, impotent and barren, those with varicose veins, headaches, boils, and diseases of every conceivable organ have left stone images, or votives, or written descriptions of their cures to adorn the ancient temple walls (Achterberg, 1985, p. 56).

Unsurprisingly, therefore, the cult of Asclepios spread widely, and by the fifth century BC his influence had extended beyond Greece into Italy and Turkey, where temples in his honour flourished. Aristotle, who was trained in the Asclepian tradition, emphasized the role of the imagination in health and illness, insisting that images, as the mediators of emotion, cause changes in bodily functions and affect both the development of disease and its cure. He regarded dream images as particularly important, claiming that they could elucidate an unsuspected illness which may have escaped waking consciousness (Boersma and Houghton, 1990).

Hippocrates was also trained in the Asclepian tradition and subsequently established a medical school which flourished until the end of the fifth century BC. He integrated medicine into the universal laws of nature as they were then conceived, thereby unifying medicine and philosophy. Accordingly, the healthy state of man and nature was considered to consist of an equivalence of basic elements, or harmony, which was an adaptation to context. Students of medicine were therefore taught to study the effects of natural cycles, such as the seasons, on health and to use all their senses to measure and define the environment. The physician, like the shaman, was therefore a diviner of natural signs and an expert in natural lore, with an awareness of the wholeness of things, who did not regard disease as an isolated phenomenon. Moreover, like the shaman, the physician recognized the power of imagination in sickness and health.

Hippocrates recognized the life force inherent in all living organisms as nature's healing power (the *vix medicatrix naturae*) and placed great emphasis on it, insisting that the physician does not heal, but only assists the healing process by creating the most favourable conditions for self-healing. He therefore viewed the physician as a servant of nature; as an attendant to the healing process, or therapist (from the Greek *therapeia* meaning attendance).

There is little doubt that the tradition of medicine established by Hippocrates was inspired by mystical vision, and it is therefore ironic that he is regarded as the father of modern medicine because in the main his views were diametrically opposed to much modern medical theory and practice. However, in the Hippocratic system there emerges for the first time the awareness that health and illness are natural biological phenomena; the reactions of an organism to its environment, lifestyle and other mundane factors rather than the work of gods and spirits. By emphasizing that health and illness can be influenced by therapeutic procedures and wise management of one's life it broke with the mystical/magical tradition of ancient medicine. In so doing it heralded a turning point in human history, when the mystic vision of the ancients became fragmented, obscured and virtually lost to Western civilization; a period when 'rational thought was emerging from the mythological dream world' (Koestler, 1984, p. 27).

This breach with ancient mysticism is largely attributable to Pythagorus, whose philosophy, ironically, is the perfect embodiment of the mystic view of the universe, integrating science, religion, mathematics, music and medicine; body, mind and spirit, in what Koestler terms 'an inspired, luminous synthesis'. However, his discovery that the pitch of a note depends on the length of the string that produces it, and that concordant intervals in the scale are produced by simple numerical ratios was epoch-making in that it reduced the ancient concept of harmony to mathematics

> It was the first successful reduction of quality to quantity, the first step towards the mathematicization of human experience – and therefore the beginnings of science (Koestler, 1984, p. 27).

Pythagorean mathematics were to prove the greatest single influence on Western thought. As Russell (1948) indicated, mathematics are the chief source of belief in external and exact truth, as well as in a super-sensible and intelligible world. As he observed, the exactness of geometry, which is not matched in the real world, suggests that all exact reasoning applies to ideal as opposed to sensible objects, and when taken further, to the belief that the objects of thought are more real than those of sense perception. In stark contrast to mysticism, therefore, it raises the status of the intellect and reduces that of intuition, sensation and feeling. However, while the Pythagoreans were aware that the symbols of mysticism and mathematics were different aspects of the same reality, this unitary awareness was rapidly lost thereafter.

Inevitably the concept of measure or ratio lost its mystical significance, becoming conceptualized as that point on a line which divides it into segments, such that the smaller is to the larger as the larger is to the whole. This measure, known as the golden mean or section, came to be imposed as an objective fact about reality and learned by mechanical conformity to teaching rather than acquired intuitively through the development of insight into the inner essence of things. Measure therefore came to denote mainly a standard of comparison with some arbitrary external standard, and as such it was disseminated through Western civilization.

Consequently knowledge came to be viewed as essentially linear, as objective fact or reality, which constitutes the only valid knowledge of the world. This idea was to have enormous implications for all subsequent thinking within the Western world. From it the West derives its notion of time as a linear sequence from the past, through the present to the future, and the idea of progress. It also derives from it an emphasis on measurement, standardization, rationality and reason, all of which involve dissection and analysis. Western man thus came to believe in an orderly linear universe that he could in time explore rationally, through reason (the possession of which sets man apart from the rest of creation) by reducing it to its constituent elements, bit by bit. Dissection and analysis have since come to characterize Western thinking and science.

The first evidence of this tendency came in the sixth century BC with the Eleatic School of philosophy. This challenged the dominant belief of the period in a unified universe of perpetual change or becoming, by arguing initially for the existence of a divine unifying principle standing above and apart from all gods and men. This devolved into a belief in one pure immutable being as the only object of knowledge and the illusoriness of all information obtained by the senses; a personal God, standing above and directing the world. God thus became external to, or other than man, and as such a fact or truth (indeed the ultimate fact or truth) and the very embodiment of Western thought.

Russell (1959, p. 56) has observed that were it not for the Greek concept of an external world revealed to the intellect but not the senses, the notion of God as it is known in the West might not have existed. However, the existence of this concept had very important consequences for Western culture in general and its medicine in particular. Fromm (1951) indicated that it led to a projection of man's personal powers onto God, which, he argued, resulted in man's alienation from himself, and separation from his most valuable powers and potentials, which is the very antithesis of magic. Furthermore, the magician's belief in his or her ability to alter consciousness at will so as to commune with and influence the forces of nature was an assault on the omnipotence of God. Therefore all practices which emphasized the development of human powers and potentials were systematically eradicated in Western culture. Sources of ancient wisdom were eclipsed as all bodies of knowledge became framed within the dominant religious traditions. Hence, by the end of the classical period of Greek history several developments in thinking had occurred which had profound and lasting influence on subsequent Western thought and overshadowed the instinctive wisdom of early man on which ancient systems of healing were based. Nevertheless statues of the Asclepian family, the caduceus symbol and the Hippocratic oath (which begins 'I swear by Apollo, the Physician, by Asclepios, by Hygiea and by Panacea and by all the Gods and Goddesses, making them my witness') have all persisted down the ages and serve as a reminder of it.

The 'last important pillar in the millenium of Greek medical pre-eminence'

(Achterberg, 1985, p. 56) was Galen, a Greek physician, anatomist and physiologist of the first century AD who, by codifying existing medical knowledge, exerted an important influence on the practice of medicine in the West throughout the Middle Ages. His system of medicine was based on the theories and practices of Hippocrates, and it incorporated understanding of the effects of imagination on health and illness. Imagery, notably that of dreams, was thought to reveal clinically important diagnostic information and to foster the development of malignancy once established. Indeed Galen anticipated modern research findings by indicating that images of sadness, terror or fright produce discrete physiological effects.

Imaginative medicine during the Middle Ages

While it is probable that many cures could also be attributed to imagination, as Achterberg (1985, p. 58) observes, it is very difficult to chronicle accurately the role of the imagination in medicine from the end of the Greek era until the Renaissance because of the influence of the Christian church, on whose authority science rested. Imagery continued to play a role in the institutionalized religions of Christianity, Judaism and Islam, which all elaborated doctrines and policies based on reason. 'It could not be otherwise, for all religions involve the notion of a spiritual universe, that cannot be verified in the physical world' (Sheikh, Kunzendorf and Sheikh, 1989), and the rituals of these religions rely heavily on imagery which is considered an effective technique in helping the faithful attain their spiritual goals. Moreover, throughout history many rich mystical traditions have co-existed with the institutionalized forms of Christianity, Judaism and Islam. The rites of Kabbalism, the Jewish mystical tradition, are heavily reliant on visual imagery, as is the Gnostic tradition of Christianity, which like Kabbalism involves visualization of ascent and descent to other worlds, and direct visionary experience of God. Meditation and visualization are also emphasized in Sufi, the mystical tradition of Islam.

However, according to Christian orthodoxy, ultimate knowledge was considered to be the preserve of God, therefore knowing too much constituted sin. All visionary and mystical traditions were therefore suspect and during the Middle Ages groups whose practices involve symbolic, magical and ascetic rituals relying on visualization, such as the Cathars, Bogomils, Albigenses, Freemasons, Kabbalists and Rosicrucians, were intensely persecuted by the Christian Church. Early Christian sects such as the Gnostics (from the Greek *gnosis* meaning knowledge) which promoted self-knowledge as the key to enlightenment and encouraged visionary experience through visualization, meditation, symbolic and magical rituals, were also stamped out by orthodox Christians within a couple of hundred years, and with such vehemence that no gnostic texts were available at first hand until 1945 when a number were rediscovered (Boot, 1993).

However, those most systematically and relentlessly purged throughout the

Middle Ages as heretics and purveyors of magic, were witches. Achterberg indicates that according to some scholars the word 'witch' signified superior knowledge or wisdom, possibly being derived from similar words meaning to prophecy or to know. She reiterates Gage's (1893) claim that they were in fact the most advanced scientists of the period, privy to healing rites preserved in secret oral traditions and shared only by initiates. Indeed, although by the fifteenth century Greek thought, language and literature had been carried to every corner of Europe, Paracelsus (1493–1541), the noted physician and founder of modern chemistry, attributed his understanding of the laws and practices of medicine to his conversations with these wise women. Consequently, most of the healing practices of the period can only be deduced from documents relating to witch trials.

Anthropologists have concluded from these documents that witches were shamanic in their regard for the unity of all things, in their attempts to use the forces of nature for healing, their knowledge of herbal lore and in their understanding of the role of the healer. This is reflected in Paracelsus' observation that 'man is his own doctor...the physician is in ourselves and in our own nature are all the things we need'. Many of the practices of witches were consistent with those of shamanism, most notably their 'flight' on broomsticks, which may be regarded as imaginative 'flights of fantasy' within the unconscious, their use of spells and drugs, and the manipulation of the imagination by way of rituals and incantations. There is little doubt that they were powerful and effective healers, but in the eyes of the Church their cures were the work of the devil, and as agents of the devil the witches were purged. Arguably, therefore, the advent and spread of Christianity effectively brought about the Dark Ages of medicine:

> The pagans (Greeks, Egyptians and Romans) had elevated the art of healing to a height it would not see again for centuries. As Christianity spread its own gospel, all that was pagan, including the pagan practice of medicine, had to fall by the wayside...the Church expunged the exquisite surgical and herbal skills of the Greeks from the roster of available treatments and substituted instead frequently brutal practices such as mortifying the flesh. This brought the practice of physical medicine to an all time low (Achterberg, 1985, p. 64).

However, as Achterberg observes, with the decline of physical medicine, imaginative medicine flourished. Indeed 'the treatments of choice specified by the early Church were medicine of the imagination in every sense: shrine cures, processions and pilgrimages to holy places, relics of the saints and martyrs' (p. 64). Healing was no longer attributed to Asclepios and his family but to saints, notably Cosmas and Damian, who became the patron saints of the healing profession throughout Western civilization. Achterberg indicates that churches dedicated to them used the method of incubatio, or incubation sleep, modelled on the divine sleep cures of the Greeks. In these the sick received diagnostic information and cures from revered healers, images of whom appeared during the twilight state between sleep and wakefulness. This practice has continued within the Christian church until the present, as has its reputation for effecting exceptional cures. Hence, she claims, 'the methods of the shamans and the wise women – healing in nonordinary reality and invoking visions of spirit guides – has been a part of Christianity since its inception. Only the names have been changed' (Achterberg, 1985, pp. 65–6).

Thus, while the heretics and witches had largely been killed off during the Middle Ages imaginative medicine continued to flourish. By the sixteenth century (the era of Paracelsus and Montaigne) the imagination was generally considered to be a powerful factor in health and illness, capable of producing diseases and curing them. Paracelsus considered it a most important tool in medicine, describing it as man's 'invisible workshop' (Hartman, 1973). However, by the end of the century the authority of the church had begun to be questioned as the discoveries of Copernicus (1473–1543) and Galileo (1564–1642) made it increasingly difficult to attribute to man the significance assigned to him in Christian theology.

Mechanistic medicine

Until the seventeenth century the aim of science was understanding and living in harmony with nature. This was radically changed by Francis Bacon (1561–1626) who asserted that science should be used to gain mastery over nature. His stance was anti-theological inasmuch as it encouraged man to sequester powers formerly attributed to God. Inevitably it brought science and religion into conflict and created a schism between the physical and spiritual realms. This was further advanced by Descartes (1596–1650) who proposed that mind and matter are fundamentally separate. This gave rise to the belief that the world could be described in terms of material objects which existed independently of human observers. This material world was considered to be assembled like a huge machine, operated by impersonal laws that could be explained in terms of the arrangement and movement of its parts, and described using simple mathematics. Descartes' world view was therefore not only mechanistic and materialistic but also analytic and reductionist in so far as he considered complex wholes as understandable in terms of their constituent parts. He extended this mechanistic model to living organisms, likening animals to clocks composed of wheels, cogs and springs, and later extended this analogy to man. To Descartes therefore, the human body was a machine; part of a perfect cosmic machine, governed, in principle at least, by mathematical laws. This view of the body as a mindless machine has governed Western medicine ever since.

His description effectively turned the human body into a clockwork and placed a distance not only between body and soul but also between the patient's complaint and the physician's eye. Within this mechanical framework pain turned into a red light and sickness into mechanical trouble. A new kind of taxonomy of diseases became possible. As minerals and plants could be classified, so diseases could be isolated and put in their place by the doctor-taxonomist. The logical framework for a new purpose in medicine had been laid (Illich, 1975, p. 112).

Subsequently the focus of medicine became disease rather than health. Diseases came to be seen as autonomous and to be spoken of as things rather than part of the life process. Increasingly the person was separated from the illness and the interest of the doctor shifted from the sick to the sickness. The practice of medicine became medical science and hospitals became laboratories for the study of disease processes rather than institutions for the care of the sick.

Newton (1643–1727) subsequently formulated the mathematical laws or mechanics which were thought to operate the cosmic machine and to give rise to all changes observable in the physical world. Hence, by the end of the seventeenth century, the holistic view of a harmonious universe in which all phenomena, including man, are interrelated and interdependent had been displaced by a clockwork model, and this subsequently guided all scientific endeavour for the next 200 years.

Over this period, the Divine was progressively eclipsed by science so that by the nineteenth century the philosopher Nietzche could justifiably declare God 'dead' in the sense that traditional meanings and values had been negated, and physical science had become the ultimate authority in Western culture. This was to have profound implications, because for the first time in human history religion was completely divorced from medicine.

2 Modern developments in imaginative medicine: psychotherapy

> The soul never thinks without a picture.
> *Aristotle*

The ethnopsychologist Holger Kalweit (1988, p. 21) has observed that 'If mankind has one thing in common it is surely the belief in the existence of a soul...This notion can be found almost without exception among all traditional peoples and cultures and indeed also in modern civilization'. Within Western civilization the idea of the soul as the vehicle of personal existence is continuous from antiquity to the present. Until the seventeenth century, the history of Western psychology consists essentially of the enumeration of doctrines concerning the soul and medicine was largely the application of knowledge concerning the soul to healing. Accordingly traditional healers made no distinction between religion and medicine. However, from the Renaissance onwards Western culture acknowledged the soul less and less, and as science displaced religion during the nineteenth century, medicine became progressively secularized and the spiritual components of disease obscured, and then ignored. With the rise of economic materialism and a mechanistic, purely object-oriented science, modern culture in the West came to look on the soul or psyche as no more than a primitive and superstitious notion without content or reality. Emphasis within medicine shifted entirely onto the physical aspects of disease as medicine became exclusively concerned with the body. Disease, whose origin could not be attributed to the physical body, was incorporated into the framework of physical science by the simple expedient of converting the soul or psyche into mind, and then into brain function, or dismissing it altogether.

The materialistic prejudice of medicine explains away the psyche as a merely epiphenomenal by-product of organic processes in the brain. Accordingly any psychic disturbance must be an organic or physical disorder which is undiscoverable only because of the insufficiency of our actual diagnostic means (Jung, 1946, p. 10).

Hence, in the view of modern Western medicine, either the body is ill or there is nothing wrong with it. Furthermore as Jung (1960, p. 344) observed, 'the modern belief in the primacy of physical explanations has led to a psychology without a psyche'. By the early twentieth century psychology, which since its origins in ancient Greece had been concerned with the study of the soul, thus became a science lacking its main subject matter. Psychopathology, formerly regarded literally as sickness of the soul, came to be seen as mental illness. A concept which Szasz (1979) claims enables human problems to be treated as part of medical science and in accordance with its principles. Similarly, psychotherapy or curing the soul, came within the remit of the 'brain sciences'.

One implication of this shift for medicine was that doctors became heir to what Frankl (1969) terms a 'medical ministry' for which they had no specialized expertise. It fell to them to wrestle with the task of reconciling the spiritual, or psychical, with the material and medical – a venture doomed to fail, as Jung (1978, p. 79) pointed out, since Western science was dismissive of all spiritual concerns. Indeed, rather than effect a reconciliation it resulted in an even greater schism, and a breakdown in the relationship between the pioneers of modern psychotherapy, Sigmund Freud and Carl Gustav Jung.

SIGMUND FREUD

Freud (1856–1939) is generally credited as being the founder of modern psychotherapy. More properly he can be thought of as the pioneer of psychological medicine inasmuch that everything embraced in his approach originated in medical science. As Jung (1966 p. 34) observes 'it bears the unmistakable imprint of the physician's consulting room – a fact which is evident not only in its terminology but also in its framework of theory'. It is also discernible in its most distinctive feature, the analyst's couch. Freudian theory and psychotherapy therefore abound with postulates which the physician has taken over from natural science. This is unsurprising, because as Fromm (1980) points out, Freud was very much a man of his time and like other nineteenth century physicians saw science as the ultimate authority. He was a self-proclaimed enemy of religion, which he viewed as an illusion preventing man from reaching maturity and independence. He described it as a universal obsessional neurosis (Jacobs, 1992). He also had a horror of the occult, by which, according to Jung (1972a, p. 173) he meant virtually everything that philosophy, religion and the emerging field of parapsychology had contributed to an understanding of the psyche. Freud wished to establish psychotherapy as a scientific discipline fully consistent with the thinking of the time. He therefore used the basic concepts of nineteenth century physics in his descriptions of psychological phenomena and subsequently 'made unjustified and mistaken claims to have established psychology on foundations similar to those of any other science, such as physics'. In claiming this Freud fooled himself as well as many of his followers (Hearnshaw, 1989, p. 157), but in the process he developed 'a model of human consciousness which dispensed with spiritual aspirations and made them disreputable' (Jackson, 1992, p. 13). The emergence of a soul-less psychology can therefore be attributed in good measure to his influence.

Freud assumed a kind of psychic energy capable of increase, diminution, displacement and discharge spread over the memory traces of ideas in much the same way as an electrical charge is distributed over the surface of a body. This circulated within a mental apparatus which he conceived as having structure. Initially he described this in two parts, conscious and unconscious, but eventually he came to view it as having three components, the id, ego and superego.

Ideas, impulses and emotions were regarded as located in specific parts of this apparatus. Changes were thought to result from movements of energy from one region to another, while actions were thought to be accompanied by a discharge of energy. Freud held that this energy existed in two forms, mobile and bound; both originating in bodily processes which he equated with sexuality. He regarded the former as characteristic of unconscious mental processes and as chaotic and unstructured, but the latter as structured, organized and characteristic of conscious mental processes. He believed that unconscious (id) impulses, ideas and emotions strive energetically to become conscious but are prevented from doing so by the action of various mechanisms which defend the conscious mind or ego from them. Accordingly, personality is a defence against these unconscious strivings and manifests in habitual stereotyped responses to situations.

Freud thus conceived of mind as a structure at war with itself, and advocated introversion, or looking inwards, as a means of achieving balance between the conscious and unconscious and resolving this conflict or dis-ease. Freudian psychotherapy therefore 'aims at an artificial introversion for the purpose of making conscious the unconscious components of the subject' (Jung 1978, p. 84). The early stages of this process consisted in putting a person in touch with the hinterland of his or her mind, and therefore can be likened to the practices of yoga, tantra and traditional magic. Indeed, Freud's role as a therapist was little different from that of the shaman. The methods he employed were remarkably similar, involving as they did evocations and interpretations of the imagination as revealed in hypnosis, fantasy, word associations, memories and, especially, dreams, which Freud considered to be of central importance, declaring them 'the royal road to the unconscious'.

> The great importance of dreams, according to Freud, was due to the entry they gave to the repressed primary areas of the mind, the 'imperishable' primitive regions, the contents of which emerged not only in dreams but in neurotic and psychotic disturbances. Freud's central hypothesis was

that there were 'no indifferent dream stimuli'. Dreams were motivated, were the expression of wishes; they had, therefore, a meaning which could be discovered. The meaning was not, however, immediately apparent, because the 'manifest' content of the dream did not directly reveal the 'latent' content. The dream 'censorship' and the processes of 'dream work' introduced disguises, condensations and distortions. Dreams, therefore, had to be interpreted, and this could be done partly by getting the dreamer to associate around the dream content, and partly by a translation of certain commonly employed dream symbols, using analogies from folklore and mythology in support. Dreams generally had several layers of meaning, the deepest stratum, Freud believed, deriving from the experiences of infancy, often from the first three years of life, and possessing sexual significance (Hearnshaw, 1989, p. 160).

Dream analysis was therefore the core of Freud's psychotherapy, but his theory of dreams was inadequate in two respects. He had no knowledge of the physiological changes that accompany dreaming, first discovered in the 1950s, or of subsequent research which suggests that the function of dreams is not merely psychological, as Freud claimed, but in part at least biological. A more serious weakness, as Hearnshaw indicates, are his canons of dream interpretation.

The accumulation of many exactly similar instances affords us the required certainty, asserted Freud. This is, of course, a logical fallacy, as it does not rule out systematic bias; and when he goes so far as to state that 'anything in a dream may mean its opposite', any hope of falsification seems to have vanished; and a theory is not scientific unless open to falsification (Hearnshaw, 1989, p. 161).

Hearnshaw concludes that while Freud did not buttress the insights afforded by dreams with convincing scientific proof, his book *The Interpretation of Dreams* is nevertheless a masterpiece. It summarized for the first time the basic principles of his theory, notably the concept of psychic reality 'a special form of existence, which must not be confounded with material reality' and of the unconscious. Jung considered Freud's achievements not only theoretical, but also practical, claiming that 'by evaluating dreams as the most important source of information concerning the unconscious processes, he gave back to mankind a tool that had seemingly been lost' (Jung, 1972, pp. 168–9).

Freud's emphasis on the unconscious has led to him being credited, quite wrongly, with having discovered it. In fact the concept of unconscious mental processes was conceived in about 1700, had become very popular by 1800 and was commonplace by 1870. At his seventieth birthday celebrations Freud admitted not having discovered or even rediscovered the unconscious, but he did claim that in psychoanalysis he had discovered and developed a method by which it could be studied. Such a claim is, of course, controvertible given the precedence of imaginative medicine.

Although uncovering the contents of the unconscious and understanding its processes was fundamental to psychoanalysis, as a method it was the very antithesis of its precursors, being (as the term suggests) explicitly reductionist and analytical as opposed to holistic, implicitly materialist and aspiritual. Freud established psychological space as a frame of reference for the structures of a 'mental apparatus' (the id, the ego and superego) which were seen as some kind of internal objects, the interactions of which explained human nature. Accordingly spatial metaphors such as depth psychology, deep unconscious and subconscious are prominent throughout Freudian theory. Although Freud described these structures as abstractions and resisted attempts to associate them with specific structures and functions of the brain, they nevertheless had all the properties of material objects. The dynamic aspects of psychotherapy, like those of Newtonian physics, therefore consist of describing how the material objects interact with one another through forces that are essentially different from matter. These forces have definite directions and can reinforce or inhibit each other, the most fundamental among them being instinctual drives, notably sexual drive or libido. 'Thus in the Freudian system the mechanisms and machineries of the mind are all driven by forces modelled after classical mechanics' (Capra, 1982a, p. 187).

The role of the therapist was to understand the workings of the mind-machine in terms of these elements, and to eliminate the obstacles to normal functioning that were considered to give rise to mental illness. Psychoanalysis is therefore primarily a diagnostic procedure, and as a treatment is only concerned with the alleviation of symptoms. It thus clearly reflects the disease model of medicine wherein health is absence of disease or pathological symptoms. Moreover, because Freud advocated the scientific ideal of objectivity he insisted that analysts should be as 'cold as surgeons' in their explorations of the mind and could 'operate' without physical intervention and minimal interaction with their clients. As a method, psychoanalysis therefore tends to be cold and impersonal and to reflect the mind–body division characteristic of medicine, neglecting the body just as emphatically as medical treatment neglects the mind. Consequently the techniques of imaginative medicine generally came to be seen as a means of treating 'psychological' as opposed to physical problems.

CARL JUNG

During the early years of the twentieth century Freud attracted a substantial following within the medical profession throughout Europe, and subsequently inspired a number of psychoanalytically orientated imaginative approaches to therapy in the USA (e.g. Reyher, 1963, 1977; Shorr, 1978, 1983; Horowitz, 1978). One of his most influential supporters was the Swiss psychiatrist Carl Gustav Jung, initially a close collaborator. However, although sharing many of Freud's views on the nature of the unconscious, the significance of dreams and other imaginative processes, Jung became increasingly critical of Freud's approach. Jung (1959) attributed the gulf between them to a difference in philosophical background, claiming that while he was steeped in philosophy, Freud had no philosophical training. As Hearnshaw (1989, p. 166) indicates 'Ideologically they were always, in fact, poles apart'.

Certainly contrasts in their approach are discernible at many levels, but the major difference between them is Jung's espousal of the magico-religious tradition. It was Freud's determination to make psychoanalysis 'an unshakeable bulwark against the black tide of mud', which is how he described occultism, that struck irrevocably at the heart of their friendship. His denial of all things spiritual or psychical was to Jung an absurdity, and an irony, given that in certain respects Freud's methods were very similar to the occult traditions he so despised. Jung insisted that 'man has, everywhere and always, spontaneously developed religious forms of expression, and the human psyche from time immemorial has been shot through with religious feelings and ideas. Whoever cannot see this aspect of the human psyche is blind, and whoever chooses to explain it away or to enlighten it away has no sense of reality' (1966, p. 140). He considered that until the religious dimension of man is given proper consideration the problem of the psyche cannot be approached and is therefore essential to any system of psychology which purports to study man. He insisted that 'a religious attitude is an element in psychic life whose importance can hardly be overrated' (1966, p. 77), claiming that he had not seen one patient over 35 years of age

> whose problem in the last resort was not that of finding a religious outlook on life. It is safe to say that every one of them fell ill because he had lost that which living religions of every age have given their followers, and none of them has been really treated who did not regain his religious outlook – this of course has nothing whatever to do with a particular creed or membership of a church (1966, p. 264).

Jung therefore considered that a truly religious attitude presupposes a healthy mind and that healing is essentially a spiritual problem. Accordingly the central thrust of his psychotherapy can be understood and described as modern man's search for his soul. It is, as Jacobi (1962) observes, a 'heilsweg' in the two-fold sense of the German word: a way of healing, and a way of salvation. It has curative power and can release psychic disturbances but also lead the individual to 'salvation' (knowledge and fulfilment of his or her own personality). It is therefore a method of both medical treatment and self-education, and of value to the sick and healthy alike.

Jung's central theoretical concerns were to map out both the structure and dynamics of the psyche, and to understand its totality as it relates to the wider environment. He conceived of the psyche as a self-regulating system comprising two antithetical but complementary spheres, the conscious and unconscious. He did not consider the latter an individual feature but collective and common, not merely to the whole of humanity, but the entire cosmos. Thus, just as physical bodies bear within their structure the marks of their evolutionary development from the lower kingdoms of nature, so, in Jung's view, the mind shows a similar line of ascent, leading Butler (1982, p. 16) to describe Jung as the Darwin of psychology.

The structure of the psyche

The structure of the psyche, according to Jung, comprises a personal unconscious beneath the conscious mind consisting of ideas, emotions and memories which have been pushed below the threshold of conscious awareness because of the individual's refusal to acknowledge them. These complexes tend to break away from the general unity and become independent or dissociated. Deeper within this level is the collective unconscious which is not individual but universal and whose contents and modes of behaviour are more or less the same in all individuals. Here reside the primordial or archaic energies which Jung termed archetypes. These are patterns of life energy which have become impressed on the psyche during the course of its evolution, thereby reflecting the life experiences of man and his predecessors, and which are shared with all humanity, present and past. As such these patterns of psychic activity are unconscious and unknowable directly, but may be interpreted as images. 'Comprehensive pictures' of the qualitative aspects of these energies are therefore provided by the symbols of visual imagery. Symbols are thus the supreme mediators between different worlds of experience, and, as Jung (1967) indicates, transformers of energy. Hence symbolism, literally that which brings together (from the Greek *sumballein* meaning to throw together), is the traditional language of the mystic, magician and poet. As Blair (1975, p. 106) observes 'The hidden order which surrounds us cannot be perceived by logic alone and we must pass over to the ships of symbolism to ride through the waters of the soul'. The energy patterns can be pictured and depicted in various ways, and personified as gods and goddesses, kings, warriors, angels and so on. Archetypal images which recur throughout fairy tales, mythology, magical, religious and mystery traditions are therefore, according to Jung, essentially metaphors for primordial experience.

> The phrase 'representations collective', which Lévy-Bruhl uses to denote the symbolic figures of the primitive view of the world, could easily be applied to the unconscious contents as well, since we are actually dealing with the same thing. Primitive tribal lore treats of archetypes that are modified in a particular way. To be sure, these archetypes are no longer the contents of the unconscious, but have already changed into conscious formulas that are taught according to tradition, generally in the form of esoteric teaching. This last is a typical mode of expression for the

transmission of collective contents originally derived from the unconscious. (Jung, 1963, pp. 53–4).

Another well-known expression of the archetype is myth and fable. But
here we are also dealing with conscious and specifically moulded forms
that have been handed on, relatively unchanged, through long periods of
time. It is thus only indirectly that the concept of the archetype fits the
representations collectives, for it properly designates the psychic content
that has as yet been subjected to no conscious treatment and so represents
an immediate, psychic actuality (Jung, 1963, pp. 53–4).

According to Jung, the unconscious can only be known indirectly through
images and symbols encountered in dreams, fantasies and visions, therefore
study of these can provide insight into the energies acting deep within the psyche.

The psyche consists essentially of images. It is a series of images in the
truest sense, not an accidental juxtaposition or sequence but a structure
that is throughout full of meaning and purpose; it is a picturing of vital
activities and just as the material of the body that is ready for life has a
need of the psyche in order to be capable of life, so the psyche presupposes the living body in order that its images may live (Jung, 1960, pp.
325–6).

Jung therefore recognized the reciprocity of mind and body, and the
mind–body unity as a dynamic life process. He also realized that imagery is a
vehicle for perceiving and experiencing this process, and that because the energies they picture are living and alive, images are similarly active and alive, and
can be interacted with. He therefore advocated exploration of these energies by
way of a process which he termed active imagination. This consists of suspension of the critical faculty, allowing emotions, fantasies and waking dream
images to emerge from the unconscious, and confronting them as if they were
objectively present. The person therefore actively interacts with these energies,
albeit within the imagination, through 'the spontaneous experiencing, envision-
ing and speaking of the configurations of existence as psychic presences'
(Hillman, 1975); that is, by personifying them as images and entering into
discourse with them. It is not merely looking passively at images as though
projected on a screen, but rather more like a play in which dialogue goes back
and forth between the personified image which has been produced spontaneously and the self which produced it. In this way information and understanding can be gained about the dynamics of the psyche. Von Franz notes that if
inner images are merely looked at, nothing happens, and that it is necessary to
enter into the process by way of personal reactions. Therefore, 'an alert, wake-
ful confrontation with the contents of the unconscious is...the very essence of
active imagination' (Von Franz, 1975, p. 112).

The dynamics of the psyche

Jung conceived of the dynamics of the psyche in terms of psychic energy or the life force, for which he adopted Freud's term libido. In the manner of Hippocrates he viewed this as play between pairs of complementary features, each of which is opposite in content and energic intensity. However, in the total system the quality of energy is constant and only its distribution variable. It follows from this that energy can be displaced, flowing from one member of a pair to its opposite, and can also be transferred from one to another by a direct act of will, in which case its mode of operation and manifestation are transformed. Displacement of energy occurs only when there is a gradient of intensity, or difference in potential, expressed psychologically by the pairs of opposites; that is, when they are unbalanced. Hence blocking of libido causes neurotic symptoms and complexes, and leads to breakdown in any pair of opposites when one side is 'emptied'.

Energy lost by consciousness in this process passes into the unconscious and activates its contents which then embark on a life of their own and erupt into consciousness, often provoking disturbances, neuroses and psychoses. Jung therefore regarded neurosis as a state of being at war with oneself, but unlike Freud he did not see this as negative, maintaining that neuroses tend towards something positive, shaking people out of their apathy. Therefore in spite of their laziness they can touch off the struggle for whole personality and health. In this sense, Jung saw order and organization arising spontaneously out of disorder and chaos.

According to Jung, the flow of psychic energy has direction, which is distinguishable as progressive or regressive movement in temporal succession. The former takes its direction from the conscious mind and the latter from the unconscious when the former fails. Progression is therefore a conscious act of will, whereas regression is unconscious. Both are necessary, transitional flows of energy. The second important quality of energy is that it moves not only forward and back but inward and outward. The specific form in which energy manifests in the psyche is the image, which is raised up by the formative power of imaginato or creative fantasy from the material of the collective unconscious. Creative action of the psyche transforms unconscious content into such images, and intuitions as appear in dreams, visions and fantasies. Thus when normal conscious energy is turned inwards it proceeds to work on the material of the unconscious. When we 'concentrate on a mental picture, it begins to stir, the image becomes enriched by details, it moves and develops...and so when we concentrate on inner pictures and when we are careful not to interrupt the natural flow of events, our unconscious will produce a series of images which makes a complete story' (Jung, 1976, p. 172). This enables the person to identify and integrate this material into consciousness and thus to become more whole or healthy. He saw the use of active imagination as a training for switching off conscious thought, thereby giving a chance for unconscious content to emerge. This he regarded as important because as long as unconscious information is not understood it keeps intruding as symptoms into consciousness. Therefore the overwhelming of the conscious by the unconscious is more likely when the latter is repressed.

From the Jungian perspective, the aim of psychological development is integration or wholeness. Therefore the conscious and unconscious have to be worked on simultaneously in order that the parts of the self which are neglected or dissociated can be rediscovered and reintegrated. Jung also recognized that as the self has a dual aspect and can be oriented either inwardly or outwardly the reality of both these inner and outer worlds also have to be reconciled. He conceived of therapy as a journey along a path of personal development towards integration or perfect health, a process which he termed individuation, and which he acknowledged as an unattainable ideal. The process of individuation thus results in 'an integration or completeness of the individual, who in this way approaches wholeness, but not perfection' (Jung, 1955, paragraph 616). Implicitly therefore he drew attention to a principle of the greatest importance: that health should be conceived not as a state but as a process of becoming healthy. More explicitly he stated that the 'goal is only important as an ideal; the essential thing is the opus which leads to a goal; that is the goal of a lifetime' (Jung, 1954, paragraph 204). The process of individuation is therefore a lifetime's task which is never completed; a 'journey upon which the individual hopefully embarks towards a destination at which he never arrives' (Storr, 1990, p. 201).

Storr (1973, p. 88) has described the conscious attitude accompanying individuation as essentially one of acceptance, of ceasing to do violence to one's own nature by repressing or over-developing any particular aspect. Jung described it as 'waiting upon God', thereby emphasizing his conviction that therapy is a spiritual journey and a religious experience.

Jung, in describing the process of individuation, of the reconciling of opposites, was calling attention to a symbolic process of healing which is of great importance.

> He recognized that man, the symbolic animal, could resolve even the deepest divisions within him upon the symbolic plane; and he invented a technique of psychotherapy by which this could be accomplished (Jacobi, 1962).

Jungian therapy

Jung described his therapeutic approach, somewhat paradoxically as both analytical and complex, as opposed to the reductive method of Freudian psychoanalysis. While the latter was concerned only with the identification and exploration of the component elements of the psyche, Jung was concerned to analyse the elements and reshape the whole. Hochheimer (1969) has therefore suggested that Jung's methods should more appropriately be described as spagyric, a term which means the equivalent of analysis-synthesis, and which derives from the Greek terms, *span* meaning to separate into component parts, and *ageirein* to assemble.

Jungian therapy essentially comprises various techniques for deliberately mobilizing active imagination. According to Jung 'what the doctor does is less a question of treatment than of developing the creative possibilities latent in the patient'. Techniques for encouraging these creative possibilities include painting and drawing fantasies, dreams and meditation upon mandalas, poetry, modelling, sculpture and dance. Much emphasis is laid on the interpretation of these imaginary products, not by the therapist as in the Freudian tradition, but by the patient in collaboration with the therapist. Indeed, Jung perceived the therapist as a fellow traveller on the journey of self-realization, indicating that 'the doctor is effective only when he himself is affected' (Jung, 1972a, p. 155). He therefore redefined the doctor–patient relationship in such a way as to become more like that between a master and disciple. He emphasized that 'the relationship between physician and patient remains personal within the frame of the impersonal professional treatment' (Jung, 1966, p. 56). In the Jungian approach the human quality of the doctor or therapist is crucial. Furthermore, in his view, no one can enlighten others while remaining in the dark about him- or herself. Accordingly the first stage in healing is for the physician to heal himself, applying to himself the system he prescribes for others.

Dreams are regarded as of particular importance in Jungian therapy because Jung regarded the dream as 'specifically the utterance of the unconscious' (1972a, p. 13). However, he disagreed with Freud's claim that the dream is a facade behind which meaning lies hidden 'a meaning already known but maliciously, so to speak, withheld from consciousness' (1972a, p. 185). For Jung the dream harbours no intent to deceive, but expresses something as best it can, although the dreamer may fail to recognize this through self-deception or lack of insight. Jung therefore helped people to understand their dream images without the application of rules, theory and dogma. He claimed that he knew of no technique that might fathom these inner processes other than by paying close attention to these images, amplifying and committing them to memory through sculpture and art. Fantasy is also highly regarded, especially that which comes to people when they are neither awake nor asleep but in a state of reverie in which judgement is suspended but consciousness not lost.

Jungian therapy as magic

Jung's therapeutic approach has many parallels with various ancient and oriental traditions that attempt to lead man to self-realization and share the common aim of achieving a point of balance or becoming centred. Indeed Jung was profoundly influenced by, and drew heavily upon them in both theory and practice. However, there are also differences, for as Von Franz (1975) observes, active imagination is not programmed but is completely individualistic. The therapist does not take on the role of expert but merely initiates the process, after which the individual undertakes the inner work alone, becoming independent of the therapist. Jung's psychotherapy thus has parallels with the magical tradition especially alchemy.

Alchemists considered inorganic matter as alive rather than dead and requiring investigation through the establishment of a relationship with it rather than by technical manipulation. They sought to establish this relationship through dreams, meditation and disciplined fantasy (*phantasia in vera non phantastica*) a process very similar to Jung's active imagination, which they described symbolically. Jung realized that the alchemists were imaging the symbolic transformation of the psyche and that they had a deep understanding of the process of psychological growth and healing he called individuation.

> What the true alchemists were working with in their retorts and crucibles was the contents of their own unconscious which they projected onto the unknown chemistry of matter. The lead which they were converting into gold, was the darkness of the unknown inner world which, through the alchemical opus, they transformed into the divine light of the Self, the gold of their divine nature (Vaughan-Lee, 1992, p. 4).

Jung therefore devoted much of his life's work to interpreting the alchemical process in the contemporary language of psychology, thereby providing access to the Western magical tradition of inner transformation.

The occultist W.E. Butler (1982) considered Jung the greatest magician of the modern age, because, as he pointed out, the aim of the genuine magician is realization of the true self and thus the truth of the world which is masked by the earthly personality. Certainly the concept of the personality (from the Greek *persona* meaning mask) as a mask of the soul is central to Jungian psychology. Jungian therapy embodies two of the most central principles of magic expressed in the maxims *gnothi se auton*, know thyself (the inscription over the entrance to the Temple of the Oracle at Delphi in Ancient Greece); and *solve et coagula*, dissolve and reform. Like magic it operates on the non-verbal level of pictures and images, accessing the subconscious mind or collective unconscious, referred to in magic and by Jung (1971) as the treasure house of eternal images, through the archaic images of its rituals and symbols, and thereby producing changes in consciousness as the psychic energy which evokes the unconscious is reinforced by primordial forces emanating from spaceless and timeless regions. The resurrection of the 'deeper self' results in regeneration and reconstitution of the personal self.

Jung's system involves several methods whereby this resurgence can be effected, just as magic involves various forms of training directed towards this end. In magic, symbolic images are chosen and used by the magician to build up the mental atmosphere which will evoke the deeper levels of the mind where archaic images and energies reside. These tend to group around certain definite nuclei or centres, similar to those which Jung termed archetypes.

Evocation of and interaction with archetypal imagery is a central feature of Jungian therapy, and in this respect Jungian methods most closely resemble those of the shamans. Drury (1979) suggests, that the collective unconscious described by Jung is the terrain of the shaman's venture inwards. It is the underworld where the shaman interacts and communes with living energies, personified as human or animal spirits, which in exactly the same manner as Jungian archetypes, act as guides to the inner world of the self and others. Jungian therapy, therefore, is very clearly within the shamanic tradition of imaginative medicine, and many of the therapeutic approaches he inspired have pronounced shamanic aspects. However, as Von Franz (1975) points out, Jungian methods differ from those of the shaman because Jung did not prescribe the images to be contemplated, or intervene in any way to guide the process of active imagination. Nor did he have a monopoly on the interpretation of dreams, as the patient participated fully in this process.

It was Jung's advocacy of both magic and religion which led to the breach in his association with Freud, and to widespread dismissal of his work as 'mere' mysticism rather than science. However, influenced by Jung, numerous scholars from various disciplines have further highlighted the links between mythology and consciousness (Progoff, 1963, 1970; Von Franz, 1974; Hillman, 1975; Lilly, 1977; Grof, 1979, 1985). Moreover, Jung's contribution to the modern development of imaginative medicine was considerable, influencing the practice of psychotherapy during the twentieth century quite appreciably, especially in Europe.

CARL HAPPICH

The influence of both Freud and Jung can be discerned in the work of Carl Happich, who presented his approach to psychotherapy in the 1930s and 1940s (Happich, 1932, 1939, 1948). He regarded the level of consciousness which seems to lie between consciousness and unconsciousness as that at which the collective unconscious can express itself through symbols. He therefore viewed 'symbolic consciousness', as he termed it, as fundamental to all creative production and the healing process, and explored the therapeutic possibilities of symbolic expression through techniques which combined knowledge of oriental traditions with contemporary 'depth' psychology. Rather than work with images produced spontaneously by a person in dreams or fantasy, Happich chose to present certain symbols which his patients were invited to explore in the context of an imaginary journey, until their meaning had been discerned. Initially they would be presented with the 'Meadow Meditation' in which they were asked to imagine themselves leaving the room and walking over fields to a meadow covered with fresh grass and flowers and to look upon it with pleasure before returning by the same route to the room and relating their experiences. This exercise would be followed by the 'Mountain Meditation' in which a person was asked to go into the countryside and slowly climb a mountain, passing through a forest and finally reaching a peak from which a wide vista can be viewed. A third exercise, the 'Chapel Meditation' involved the person imagining passing through a grove and reaching a chapel which he or she enters and remains in for some time. Finally the person was invited to imagine sitting on a bench by a fountain listening to the murmur of water.

It was Happich's view that every person retains within the psyche an active and creative 'child' and that the realm of this child is revealed through visualization of the meadow, a symbol which initiates and clarifies other symbols related to this psychic realm. 'These self-crystallized symbols are unmediated expressions of the individual's adaptation to the realm of the 'child' within the psyche' (Kretschmer, 1969, p. 220), and could be used diagnostically.

> A healthy man will have a satisfying experience of a meadow in the flush of spring. He will populate the meadow with children or with the form of an agreeable woman. He will, perhaps, pick flowers and so on. In this way, the meditator discovers a symbolic representation of his psychic condition. The psychically ill find it impossible to visualize a fresh meadow and during meditation cannot find one or the meadow may be seen as wilted or composed of a single stump, or all sorts of disturbing, negative symbols may be scattered around. From such manifestations of illness one gains a diagnosis which must be translated into a therapy. Often, the meditation must be repeated many times until the crippling effects of the fundamental psychic problem are undone and the meditation can proceed normally (Kretschmer, 1969, pp. 221–2).

Climbing the mountain was similarly interpreted by Happich as symbolizing a person's movement towards the goal of psychic freedom, with passage through a forest on the way up representing the dark fearful side of his nature with which he needs to be reconciled.

Like Jung, Happich emphasized the importance of the religious factor in human life, believing that man had to address these features in order to be really healthy and psychically free. The chapel was therefore regarded as a symbol of the innermost area of the psyche where the person faces the central issues of human life.

Moreover, like Jung, Happich also made use of mandalas in his 'Design Meditation' during which patients were directed to identify psychically with the symbols inherent in the mandala and to integrate its meaning with their psychic life.

However, unlike Jung, Happich was to remain a fairly minor figure in the history of imaginative medicine, because in spite of his efforts to promote his techniques within medicine, physicians showed no interest in them. Kretschmer claims that his importance lies in having disseminated imaginative techniques among theologians.

ROBERT DESOILLE

The emphasis in the work of the Frenchman Robert Desoille is of more conventional depth psychology, although he regarded religious sensitivity as the highest psychic state as did Happich. Desoille suggested that when journeying through the realms of the imagination individuals can relate to their personal symbols and can discover in it ways of dealing with the problems of their lives. He claimed that by psychically wandering wherever they choose and by any means, patients encounter various symbolic forms manifested by the personal and collective unconscious. They can learn to control and overcome fear of this archetypal imagery within themselves, and in so doing can comprehend and resolve their personal conflicts within the larger context of man's inherent problems.

Desoille therefore advocated the therapeutic use of the 'waking dream' or 'directed daydream' (Desoille, 1945, 1965). In this approach the person journeys in the imagination, relating psychic experiences and reactions to the therapist, who as the psychological scene is presented, suggests to the client a symbolic means of changing his or her situation by images of ascent or descent. In so doing he was reiterating a procedure learned from his teacher Eugene Caslant, who taught his patients to ascend and descend from one imaginary level to another by evoking such images as a ladder, staircase or flying chariot. The therapist therefore does not suggest the whole fantasy but directs and controls it by offering symbols which can serve as points of crystallization for the fantasy. In this way 'the patient is led to the psychological execution of what Goethe poetically described as the way 'from heaven through the world to hell'. In other words, he penetrates through the patient's whole psychic report and provides symbolic expressions of inherent libidinal tendencies which motivate men on various psychic levels' (Kretschmer, 1969, p. 224).

Desoille's method bears the hallmark of psychoanalysis inasmuch as its symbols embody Freudian conceptions of the dynamics of mind. However, as Kretschmer indicates, unlike psychoanalysis where the motivational or libidinal conflict is resolved by the therapist, it requires the patient to uncover within himself the basic roots of the conflict. Unlike psychoanalysis it does not try to penetrate the psychic situation through conversation. 'It is a healing process which seeks the maximum transcendence of psychic limitations through symbolic ascensions and descensions' (Kretschmer, 1969, p. 225).

WALTER FREDERKING

Using a method which he called 'deep relaxation and symbolism', Walter Frederking (1948) also attempted to stimulate the unconscious to spontaneous productions of various kinds. His patients were encouraged to engage in fantasy during progressive physical relaxation and to describe their experiences and discoveries as they progressed from unclear visions to increasingly clearer productions of a kind of 'symbolic strip thought' (Kretschmer, 1969). This symbolic thought, which Frederking considered to have a significance similar to dream life, was allowed to flow by, with the patient as both playwright and actors. In this way, Frederking believed the person could directly confront the contents of his or her personal unconscious and relate them directly and dramatically to psychic problems. He claimed this meeting with generally unrecognized aspects of oneself brings about a healing through various transforming symbols. 'In dreams and symbols man is led through every sphere of the psyche, during which the forms of the psychic force are able to restore themselves without the use of other means and deep-going transformations are effected' (cited by Kretschmer, 1969, p. 225).

FRIEDRICH MAUZ

Friedrich Mauz (1948) used a related method with psychotic patients. By way of monologue he depicted the patient in representative scenes from childhood, the aim being to unlock and enliven suppressed emotions so that a meaningful dialogue could later emerge. He also led patients to an imaginary meadow infused with symbols which he believed would awaken positive feelings and meanings in the person, and enable them to contact their feelings and the world around them. He claimed that the creative power which flows from these symbols and feelings aids in closing the breach in the patient's personality, thereby effecting healing. Mauz identified several important principles of his approach. Essentially he regarded the symbolic scene as the effector of therapy, but 'only if it is experienced as real and actual', and if 'the therapist mixes himself into a common solution with the patient'. The latter is achieved by the therapist meditating on the patient, allowing himself to be 'caught up by formulations of their psychic power'. This he claimed 'is the mystical unity between the therapist and the sick'. For Mauz, therefore, 'the simple human relationship' was the highest principle of therapy; an idea, which as Kretschmer observes, is far removed from that of contemporary scientific medicine, but of central importance within traditional imaginative medicine.

ONEIROTHERAPIES

Hanscarl Leuner (1977, 1978, 1984) developed guided affective imagery along similar lines to those methods outlined above. Patients were invited to enter and explore a series of 10 predetermined scenes representing major conflict areas in life (the first of which is a meadow) and to provide the therapist with a commentary on the experience. Extended visual fantasies with a narrative commentary are also a feature of Fretigny and Virel's (1968) oneirodrama, which is initiated by certain standard symbolic scenes and preceded by relaxation procedures. Sheikh and Jordan (1983) observe that all of these dream or waking dream therapies, which collectively they term oneirotherapy (from the Greek *oneiros* meaning sleep) rest on the belief that the symbolism inherent in visual imagery constitutes an affective language that expresses unconscious motives without fully imposing them on conscious recognition. Therefore, it is assumed that the participant will show less resistance to the expression of underlying motives. They also note that in general these methods have been reported to be effective in uncovering the structural details of the client's personality, in discovering the nature of affective trauma, and in quickly ameliorating the symptoms. They note that Fretigny and Virel also claim other advantages of such an approach: notably its suitability for use with both relatively unsophisticated persons and those prone to rationalization.

ROBERTO ASSAGIOLI

The psychoanalytically trained Italian psychiatrist Roberto Assagioli also viewed the unconscious as a source of wisdom and healing potential and believed that people should be sufficiently in communication with the deep forces within their psyche to be able to use them, rather than be used by them. Like Jung, he considered that Freudian interpretation of unconscious imagery introduces an undesirable passive element into the therapeutic relationship. He therefore used guided imagery, day dreams or symbols as a means of allowing his patients to mediate between conscious and unconscious material themselves. He conceived of symbols as 'containers' of meaning, and therefore as transformers and conductors, or channels, of psychic energies. For Assagioli as for Jung, wholeness or health requires the integration of imagination, intuition and inspiration with rational, conscious processes. It is psychosynthesis, a bringing together of different modes of consciousness. Like Jung, Assagioli was greatly influenced by oriental mysticism, and his psychosynthesis, a system of therapy expounded and developed in the 1920s and subsequently, draws heavily on its practices. He uses meditational and mystical techniques in the development of imagination and intuition, with the aim of integrating all aspects of the self.

Although influenced by Jung, Assagioli went further than him in distinguishing between the collective unconscious and what he termed the higher or transpersonal self. One way of conceiving this distinction might be to consider the former as below or underneath consciousness and the latter as above it, in a manner analagous to the underworld and heavens of the shaman. The underworld of the collective unconscious is essentially the domain of archetypal energies which may be differentiated and represented symbolically or imaginatively as gods or guides in various forms. Whereas the heavens occupy an undifferentiated frequency domain beyond such conceptionalization which can only be experienced directly. Assagioli considered that psychoanalysis was unjustified in limiting its explorations to the 'underworld' of the unconscious and that the regions of the middle and higher unconscious should likewise be explored.

In that way we shall discover in ourselves hitherto unknown abilities, our true vocations, our higher potentialities which seek to express themselves, but which we often repel and repress through lack of understanding, through prejudice or fear. We shall also discover the immense reserve of undifferentiated psychic energy latent in every one of us; that is, the plastic part of our unconscious which lies at our disposal, empowering us with an unlimited capacity to learn and to create (Assagioli, 1991b, p. 125).

A similar distinction between the world of spirits and the world of spirit is frequently encountered in religious and mystical traditions, notably those of the East which strive towards union with and direct experience of the ultimate reality or universal mind. These emphasize that true seeing or direct perception of reality involves 'pure' consciousness, a nothingness or emptiness variously termed Brahman, Atman, the universal Tao, and described in Buddhism as 'the clear light of the void', or undifferentiated, uncoloured light which is encountered by looking inwards to the centre of one's being. These traditions all assert that this realm of consciousness is beyond all forms and appearances, albeit that from which all such forms and appearances derive. Meditation or concentration on images and symbols is therefore a means to this end, which ultimately must be transcended. By differentiating the primitive, archaic contents of the collective unconscious from the 'superconscious', Assagioli was able to make subtle distinctions between the various kinds of psychic experience in a manner more fully consistent with ancient and oriental traditions, and to embrace mysticism and spirituality even more forcefully than Jung.

The goal of his therapy was not only to explicate these various levels of awareness but by thorough exploration of them to reconstruct the total personality, shifting it to a new centre through examination of its fundamental core, and thus enhancing the personal and spiritual potential. Like Jung, he considered that this process could be undertaken alone but is accomplished more easily with the help of another.

What has to be achieved is to expand the personal consciousness into that of the self; to reach up, following the thread or ray to the star; to unite the lower with the higher self. But this, which is so easily expressed in words, is in reality a tremendous undertaking. It constitutes a magnificent endeavour, but certainly a long and arduous one, and not everybody is ready for it. But between the starting point in the lowlands of our ordinary consciousness and the shining peak of self-realization there are intermediate phases, plateaus at various altitudes on which a man may rest or even make his abode, if his lack of strength precludes or his will does not choose a further ascent. In favourable cases the ascent takes place to some extent spontaneously through a process of natural inner growth, fostered by the manifold experiences of life; but often the process is very slow. In all cases, however, it can be considerably accelerated by our deliberate conscious action and the use of appropriate active techniques (Assagioli, 1991b, pp. 127–8).

Imaginative methods are among many used to this end by Assagioli, who viewed every element of images as representing, at one level or another, a personality trait, albeit distorted, displaced or projected. He encouraged identification with all aspects of the image as a means of assimilating repressed or otherwise dissociated material into a new construction of the self.

BEHAVIOURISM

The impact of behaviourism

The publication of several books in English by Assagioli (1965, 1967, 1975, 1991a,b) helped to draw attention to the techniques of imaginative medicine. These had been disseminated widely throughout Europe in the early decades of the twentieth century by clinicians influenced by Freud and Jung, but had been virtually ignored within the field of psychological medicine in Britain and North America. This was because by the early twentieth century psychology no longer concerned itself with subjective experience of any kind. By this time all thinking was essentially analytic, reductionist, objective and positivistic in the sense that the only valid knowledge was held to be scientific knowledge or positive fact which is objectively verifiable. Under the influence of positivism, attempts were made to elevate psychology to the status of an objective natural science, and in order for this to be accomplished it was deemed necessary for it to adopt the methods and principles of physics, which was concerned with the properties of matter, and in the tradition of Cartesian–Newtonian science, was the standard for scientific rigour and objectivity. This demanded a radical change in both the subject matter and methods of psychology which throughout its history had been predominantly concerned with exploration of consciousness by way of subjective introspection. The basic premise of the scientific research tradition is that ultimate reality can only be known by way of 'objective consciousness' cleansed of all subjective distortion and all personal involvement, and that what emerges from this state qualifies as valid knowledge or fact. Scientific method therefore rejects all but objective or positive fact. Unfortunately for psychology. 'No experiences, ordinary, everyday, usual or unusual, whether impressions, ideas, dreams, visions, memories, strange, bizarre, familiar, weird, psychotic or sane, are objective facts' (Laing, 1983, p. 9). Hence, in trying to gain acceptance as a *bona fide* science since the early twentieth century, psychology has tried to distance itself from the 'irrational' aspects of its subject matter. It reconciled the apparent incompatibility of science and the psyche by denying the existence of the latter and conceiving of man solely in terms of his objective behaviour. Psychology thus became the scientific analysis of behaviour.

This 'behaviourism' as developed predominantly by American theorists, viewed man as a complex machine responding to various environmental stimuli by way of conditioned reflexes. Adopting a suitably clockwork metaphor it set itself the task of finding out how man 'ticks', without any reference to mind, much less soul or spirit, only to the brain, which as a physical entity was legitimately part of the cosmic machine. Its basic principle was that complex phenomena could be reduced to combinations of simple stimulus–response patterns, which were seen as adequate explanations for all human endeavour including religion, art and science. The attempt to understand man in what Koestler (1976) termed 'slot-machine mechanics' implied a rigorous causal relationship which would allow psychology to predict the response for any given stimulus and conversely to specify the stimulus for a given response.

Behaviour therapy

The 'mindless' approach of behaviourism, was perceived by academic psychologists as more consistent with the aims and methods of science and it overtook the psychologies of Freud and Jung. Subsequently it dominated the discipline for most of the first half of the twentieth century, reaching the peak of its ascendency during the 1950s at the height of the machine age.

When viewed against the history of medicine this 'mindless' approach is quite aberrant, for as Siegel (1986, p. 65) indicates, 'in Western practice since its beginnings in the work of Hippocrates the need to operate through the patient's mind has always been recognized'. Its effect on the practice of imaginative medicine was considerable because there is little or no place for the imagination in a universe of cogs and wheels, where man is simply a machine part. Holistic approaches to healing were supplanted by what Kaptehuk and Croucher (1986) have described as 'linear medicine' which focuses on probing, detecting, isolating, controlling and usually destroying 'problems' which are seen as invasions, defects or aberrations, quite separate from the person. Consistent with its mechanistic orientation twentieth century medicine has become progressively more concerned with engineering of various kinds (genetic, biochemical and structural) and has settled for repairing, removing or replacing those parts it cannot as yet more successfully engineer. Psychological medicine also concerned itself with engineering. In the wake of behaviourism which viewed psychological disorder as learned maladaptive behaviour patterns, psychotherapy was substituted with behaviour therapy, the goal of which is to rectify deviant behaviour patterns and restore the individual to normal functioning.

Even so, imaginal methods have not been completely obliterated in behaviour therapy, and many behavioural approaches serve to demonstrate that images are powerful stimuli which elicit emotional responses. Procedures such as systematic desensitization and emotional flooding, (Wolpe, 1969, 1977) employ imagery in conjunction with relaxation in the modification of phobic behaviour, and in attempts to change or reduce inappropriate or exaggerated responses to stress. Indeed as Lazarus (1966) states, 'a prerequisite for effective application of desensitization is the ability to conjure up reasonably vivid images'.

Systematic desensitization

Systematic desensitization, sometimes referred to as the method of reciprocal inhibition, is the most widely used of all behaviour modification techniques for the amelioration of emotional problems. It has been applied extensively and most successfully in the treatment of irrational fears or phobias and expanded to deal with a great variety of other symptomatic patterns associated with neurotic disturbance.

Initially it involves careful analysis of the nature of the phobia and the range of situations in which the phobic individual experiences anxiety. A hierarchy or sequence of different images relating to the feared event or object is then constructed, ranging from the least to the most frightening. The person is then encouraged to engage in progressive relaxation and while relaxed is confronted progressively with items in the hierarchy. In theory as each image is presented to a deeply relaxed person it loses a certain increment of its associated anxiety.

> A man who is afraid to ride on a bus, for example, might begin using the fact that the least frightening level is just to think at home of the possibility that he may have to ride on a bus. This arouses a moderate amount of anxiety. The next most frightening image is going out of the house and walking toward the bus stop. Next in order might be the thought of waiting at the bus stop and watching the bus approach. Then would come actually having to step aboard the bus and pay the fare. By constructing such a hierarchy of increasingly frightening scenes the individual pinpoints the exact sequence of fearfulness and then systematically eliminates the anxieties associated with each element in the total picture (Singer, 1975, p. 222–3).

In a variation of this procedure, the relaxed person is encouraged not only to produce the frightening images but to balance them with pleasant images.

As Singer notes, the entire method critically depends on the private imagery of the individual. In effect the therapist merely establishes conditions of relaxation and a systematic way for the patient to engage in the imagery. Essentially the images or the responses that will be desensitized are developed by the patient and are completely under his or her control.

> Since the key feature of the treatment is the patient's ability to produce imagery and to carry out, in the presence of the therapist, the day dream about various events in his life, the effect of the treatment is in part a testimonial to the great human capacity for producing fantasy material with the power to modify behaviour. So in a curious way, we come full circle. The behaviourists, who have been most critical of the emphasis by psychoanalysts and humanists on private experience and internal events in the personality, have ended up developing a treatment method that is particularly effective because it relies extensively on the imaging capacities of the patient (Singer, 1975, p. 223).

Aversion therapy

An approach employed by behaviour therapists in the treatment of alcohol and drug abuse, sexual deviation and antisocial behaviours has been to provide the patient with an extremely unpleasant or negative experience when he or she actively participates in the undesired behaviour. Electric shock and nausea-producing drugs have been used widely in the treatment of homosexuality, alcohol and drug abuse and sexual fetishes. However, as adminstration of these is often hazardous and complex, a number of behaviour modification therapists have now moved towards using the patient's own imaging capacities rather than external agents to provide a repellent experience for those who are trying to control unwanted behaviour. The covert desensitization method developed by Joseph Cautela (1967, 1993) might work as follows:

> A young man who is attempting to control a drinking habit may be encouraged to imagine himself going into a bar and asking for a drink. As he leans his elbow on the bar, he realizes he is immersing it in a pool of green vomit. In disgust, he withdraws his arm, only to realize that there is vomit all over the floor at his feet, and the stench is rising slowly around him. The bartender hands him a glass of liquor, but almost immediately he himself becomes sick and vomits over it; enveloped in the smell and seeing particles of half-digested food spraying all over his drink and hands as he stands there at the bar (Singer, 1975, p. 226).

Similar principles have been utilized in procedures developed by Kolvin (1967) and Marks and Gelder (1967). Stampfl and Lewis (1967) have developed a highly controversial 'implosive therapy' in which, rather than the patient forming suggested images in a state of calm relaxation, the therapist uses images to create a situation of intense anxiety, hoping thereby to 'implode' away symptom formation. The therapist therefore presents the patient with his or her worst imaginings surrounding an event or situation, the assumption being that if the patient imagines the worst and nothing happens, the tendency to associate fear with this image in subsequent confrontations will be reduced. Horowitz (1970, p. 308) observes, implosive therapy rests partly on shock value.

> Thus, for example, the therapist may tell a person with a rat phobia to image a rat touching them, running across their hand, biting them on the arm, piercing them viciously, devouring their eyes, and jumping down their mouths to destroy internal organs (Hogan and Kircher, 1967).

HUMANISTIC PSYCHOLOGY

Nevertheless, irrespective of whether man is viewed literally or metaphorically as a machine the net result is that he is reduced to something less than human, and, as Jung (1959) observed, 'Man does not stand forever his nullification'. During the 1950s a growing number of psychologists, especially in America, refused to view man as a machine, and attempted a fully human alternative to the mechanistic view of man prevalent within Western psychology. Their concerns, focusing as they did on the individual as a perceiver and interpreter of himself and his world and a determiner of his own behaviour, represented a return to fundamental questions regarding the nature and development of the human self, psyche or soul, and reinstated these as legitimate questions for psychology. What came to be known as humanistic psychology addressed itself to spiritual human concerns and devising new methods with which to study the significant problems of man rather than insignificant problems which fitted the so-called scientific method. These methods included a number of different therapies (Graham, 1986), all of which focused attention on consciousness, subjective experience, feelings, imagination, dreams, fantasy, personal responsibility, powers and potentials. Many, influenced by the practices of imaginative medicine in Europe and the East, developed novel imaginative methods.

Gestalt therapy

One of the most influential was Gestalt therapy, which was first demonstrated in America during the 1960s by its originator Frederick (Fritz) Perls (1893–1970), a German psychiatrist. Although originally trained in the psychoanalytic school, Perls became progressively alienated from it, and began to challenge Freudian theory and practice during the 1940s, when he began to develop an eclectic approach to therapy. Among many important influences on Perls during the 1950s were Eastern meditative traditions, notably Zen Buddhism and psychodrama. The latter was a psychotherapeutic approach developed by a contemporary of Freud, the Viennese psychiatrist Jacob Moreno, which had considerable impact in North America where Perls had been resident since 1946.

In developing psychodrama, Moreno was seeking an alternative to the predominantly verbal approach of orthodox psychoanalysis that facilitated psychological healing through powerful emotional release or catharsis. In psychodrama a principal actor or protagonist dramatizes his or her problems and conflicts in the company of several auxiliaries under the direction of a therapist, who assumes overall responsibility for the ensuing drama, and employs a number of imaginative techniques in facilitating the dramatic process. These methods utilizing imagination, role playing, play acting and play in general were subsequently widely adopted by many therapists, including Perls, who recognized their value in the exploration of fantasy.

We can make use in therapy of fantasizing and all its increasing states of intensity towards actuality – a verbalized fantasy, or one which is written down, or one which is acted out as psychodrama (Perls, 1976, p. 86).

Like Jung, Perls saw the importance of exploring everyday fantasy, recognizing that its imagery reveals a hidden reality which can be discovered and understood. The more so if the fantasy is enacted, enabling an individual to identify his or her feelings, perceptions and responses to it. He therefore encouraged his clients to imagine and explore a symbol or situation as fully as possible, and to recognize the aspects of themselves they had projected in it, or which were revealed by their resistance to so doing. They were frequently invited to re-enact their fantasies so as to identify with and take responsibility for every aspect of their creation. Perls termed this form of dramatization, monotherapy. He claimed that by requiring a person to create and enact his or her own stage, characters, props and dialogue and to direct and orchestrate every performance 'monotherapy thus avoids the contamination of the precepts of others, which are usually present in ordinary psychodrama' (Perls, 1976, p. 86).

By working with his clients 'centre-stage', as it were, in front of an audience, Perls dispensed with most of the elements of psychodramatic enactment, requiring them to play all of the parts of the drama themselves, either by acting each role (including those of the props) in turn, or by conducting dialogue between these elements, whether animate or not. For this purpose the 'empty chair technique', which is perhaps the best-known feature of Gestalt therapy, was developed. This requires a person to confront directly any element of the fantasy by projecting it on to a vacant chair and conducting an imaginary conversation with it, during the course of which the person acts out both sides of the dialogue, alternating chairs in order to do so. The imaginary occupant of the chair might be an aspect of the self typically unexpressed in a given situation (the repressed self) which Perls labelled the underdog, or other aspects of the personality, such as real or fantastical persons, creatures or objects, indeed anything the person imagines. The idea being that by bringing these features into the open the person may be able to identify and integrate the diffuse or dissociated parts of him/herself and achieve a personal synthesis or gestalt, an individual pattern or whole, synonymous with health. A related technique requires clients to shuttle or alternate between the manifest content of a fantasy and its associated imagery, in an attempt to help them understand its symbolic significance and to sharpen awareness by providing them with a clearer sense of the relationships in their behaviour. Perls employed the same method in working with dreams which he regarded as existential messengers conveying vital information necessary for the maintenance of psychological health, and with intrapsychic and interpersonal conflicts.

Using Gestalt therapy, Perls demonstrated that imagery is a rich source of information about the self and that there is no limit to the kinds of imagery that can be created and used effectively in therapy. In addition to the richness and variety of imagery he also highlighted a diversity of methods by which these images may be accessed and explored.

The impact of his approach on the development of humanistic psychotherapy has been enormous. Gestalt ideas and practices have also been assimilated directly and indirectly into other psychotherapeutic approaches. Indeed, 'there are signs that Gestalt therapy is being absorbed, as if by osmosis, into the psychotherapeutic mainstream, without recognition or acknowledgement of its contributions' (Miller, 1989, p. 23). Certainly it would not be possible to list here all the various contributors to the literature and practice of psychotherapy and counselling who have been influenced by it. Clarkson and MacKewn (1993, p. 174) observe that psychotherapists and counsellors of many orientations have integrated ideas that originated with or were popularized by Perls. Ideas 'now so thoroughly accepted that it is hard to conceive just how radical they were at the time'.

As they indicate, the dissemination of Perls' influence owes much to his itinerant lifestyle and the fact that he was extremely energetic in his attempts to establish Gestalt as an independent school of psychotherapy. It now flourishes as such throughout North America, Europe, Scandinavia, Russia and Japan, and in many of these countries it has been integrated into health care provision in medical and psychiatric settings, within education and social work and private practice. It is also used in organizational and consultancy work in the USA and Britain (Nevis, 1992; Clark and Fraser, 1987; Clarkson and Shaw, 1992).

Perls drew wide public attention to Gestalt therapy, presenting innumerable workshop demonstrations, accounts and transcripts of which were published by him (Perls, 1969, 1973, 1976) and others (Fagan and Shepherd, 1971; Shepard, 1976; Stevens, 1977) and which were the subject of numerous films and video recordings, and much media coverage. He attempted to simplify the theory on which his methods were based for a wide general readership (Perls, 1969, 1976), often coining punchy and incisive phrases which became popular slogans of the period.

THE NEW AGE

A major factor in the dissemination of Gestalt therapy was the zeitgeist of the 1960s and early 1970s. The historian Theodore Roszak (1970) indicates that prior to the mid-twentieth century science had generally been viewed as an unquestionable social good, being associated in the popular mind with progress, the promise of affluence, longevity and health. It was not anticipated that science might generate its own characteristic problems, nor that as a result of its processes man might find his existence more precarious and meaningless. World War II, which was fought by means of science and technology (generating rapid acceleration in both) together with rapid social and cultural change, had done much to alert people to the possibly undesirable consequences of scientific progress. The possibility of science becoming a tool for world domination was given greater emphasis by the cold war existing between the major world powers, Russia and the USA, and the 'space race', in which Russia nosed ahead of her great rival, the USA, with the launch of the Sputnik satellite in 1957.

Moreover, the scientific 'rape of the earth' predicted several centuries earlier by Frances Bacon was occurring on an unprecedented scale, and the exhaustion of natural resources, extinction of plant and animal species, and pollution, all testified to man's growing alienation from other species and the environment. The American Professor of Psychology, Abraham Maslow, observed that science had come to a kind of literal dead end, and could increasingly be seen as a threat or danger to mankind, or at least to its highest and most noble aspirations. He suggested that people were increasingly aware 'that science besmirches and depresses, that it tears things apart rather than integrating them, thereby killing rather than creating' (Maslow, 1968, p. viii). Another psychologist Viktor Frankl (1969) suggested that in presenting man as a mindless machine, psychology had played a part in augmenting and supporting the mass dehumanization of the era.

Science and psychology both came under increasing suspicion throughout this time and a variety of issues (nuclear power and weapons, uranium mining, pollution, conservation, animal and human rights) all became vehicles for protest. The main thrust of opposition was, however, against the arms race and war. Protest was nowhere more vocal than among young people, particularly students in American colleges and universities, many of whom faced draft into the armed forces engaged in fighting the bitter and futile war in Vietnam. Frankl observed that these students were experiencing a sense of emptiness and meaninglessness. They were distasteful of the way scientific findings were being presented to them, and the mechanistic and reductionist view of man they implied. These feelings were no doubt heightened by the disinclination of many to become dispensable cogs in the American war machine. However, Roszak suggests that the paramount struggle of the young was not against war *per se* but against the dehumanizing and alienating values of science and technocracy, that system more highly developed in America than in any other society, by which government rests on technical expertise and scientific forms of knowledge. Students urged their contemporaries to 'drop out' of this lethal culture, to turn away from science and back to nature, thereby earning the 'flower power' label with which the media dubbed the movement.

Despite much trivialization and distortion by the media, the rejection of scientific culture by the young represented perhaps the most significant and widespread social and intellectual revolution in Western culture since the seventeenth century. Tart (1975) suggests that while the causes of this rejection of science were complex and varied, a basic cause of the radical disaffiliation of youth from mainstream Western society during the 1960s and 1970s was the widespread use of drugs and psychedelics, and the fact that the visionary and spiritual experiences, and altered states of consciousness associated with them were almost totally ignored by orthodox science. Much drug use had been inspired by Aldous Huxley, a student of Mayahana Buddhism and an advocate of psychotrophic drugs as a means of enhancing and systematically exploring consciousness or 'inner space'. His writings, most notably *The Doors of*

Perception (Huxley, 1954), were very influential in stimulating interest in mystical experience. Finding that science had no place for this, many of the young turned their attention to religious and spiritual traditions that did. Drury (1979) observes that this effect is clearly reflected in the popular music of the period in which spiritual, mystical and visionary themes abound. This was further accentuated in the late 1960s when the Beatles, the most popular musicians of the time, made a much publicized spiritual pilgrimage to India and subsequently adopted as their spiritual master the Maharishi Mahesh Yogi and his practice of transcendental meditation. In their wake countless young people made their way east, among them a number of scientists, including the Harvard psychologist Richard Alpert, who later returned to the West as Baba Ram Dass to promote yoga, meditation and other techniques for expanding consciousness (Dass, 1978). There was a complementary East–West movement, albeit on a far smaller scale, first evident in the increased flow of literature from the East in the 1960s. This was followed during the 1970s by the migration West of several gurus, notably Maharaj Ji and Maharishi Mahesh Yogi, and in the 1980s by Bhagwan Shree Rajneesh, all of whom disseminated techniques of meditation, spiritual development and heightened awareness.

The growing fascination with these subjects was also reflected in an upsurgence of interest in ancient traditions and those of other cultures. Ancient Hindu texts such as the *Bhagavad Gita* were translated into English (Prabhupado, 1968), and astonishingly the *Bardo Thodol*, or *Tibetan Book of The Dead* (Evans-Wentz, 1976) and the *I Ching* (Wilhelm 1978) became best-sellers in the USA. Interest in the spiritual traditions of the East led to the names of writers such as T. Suzuki, Idries Shah, Gurdjieff, Swami Nikhilananda and Krishnamurti becoming familiar in the West as their books, and books about them, found their way onto more and more bookshelves. Zen Buddhism, which had been popularized in the novels of Jack Kerouac and Allen Ginsberg in the 1950s, was further promoted during the 1960s by Alan Watts and T. Suzuki, and subsequently in Pirsig's best-selling novel *Zen and the Art of Motorcycle Maintenance* (1974). Books by Western interpreters of Eastern traditions such as Lama Govinda, Mircea Eliade, Alan Watts, Ram Dass, Christmas Humphreys, Karlfried Durckheim and Christopher Isherwood also became popular. In addition the practice of these alternative disciplines flourished as more and more people explored Buddhism, Zen, Sufi, Yoga, Taoism and various forms of meditation. According to a Gallup poll published in *Newsweek* magazine on 6 September 1976, no less than five million Americans practised yoga, six million meditated regularly, and two million were deeply involved in oriental religion at that time.

THE OCCULT REVIVAL

There was also a widespread renewal of interest in the occult at this time, which Roszak (1975) interprets as an attempt to bring myth, magic and mystery back into twentieth century living and to return to the visionary origins of Western culture. Books by contemporary occultists such as Dion Fortune, W.E. Butler, Israel Regardie proliferated. The teachings of the highly eclectic occultist, Giorgi Gurdjieff, who had died in 1949, were widely disseminated by teachers such as Pietr Ouspensky, A.R. Orage, Thomas and Olga de Hartmann (Webb, 1980), in the writings of Peters (1964, 1965, 1978) and Anderson (1962, 1969), and by the publication during the 1970s of the major works of Gurdjieff (1974, 1976) and his autobiography (1978), which later became the subject of a feature film. Groups of followers flourished worldwide, as did various movements associated with his teachings and methods, including Arica, a psychotherapeutic approach developed by Oscar Ichazo.

Gurdjieff's teachings were undoubtedly influential in stimulating research into altered states of consciousness, including that of Lilly (1973) and Grof (1979, 1992). Both of whom claim that certain drugs, notably psychedelic drugs used in shamanic ritual, circumvent what Huxley (1954) termed the 'reducing valve of ordinary consciousness', enabling direct perception of non-ordinary reality and exploration of the realms of the unconscious.

The growing use of psychedelic drugs further stimulated interest in the magical practices of which, traditionally, it is a feature. Ostensibly at least, an attempt to investigate scientifically the relationship between drug use and magical consciousness gave rise to one of the most remarkable visionary movements of the era, that surrounding Carlos Castaneda.

Carlos Castaneda

In the early 1960s, Castaneda, an American anthropology student was awarded a doctorate degree. His thesis was an account of how he had developed visionary insight into the nature of the universe through his 12 year apprenticeship in sorcery to the Yaqui Indian sorcerer, shaman, or brujo Don Juan Matus. It was subsequently published, virtually unaltered, in 1968 and reprinted in 1970 under the title *The Teachings of Don Juan: a Yaqui Way of Knowledge*. Not only did it become an international best-seller but gained a cult following which was not confined to a general lay readership. Despite the fact that the elusive Don Juan could not be found outside the book of teachings attributed to him he was included among other modern mystics and sages in Anne Bancroft's (1978) book of that name. Elsewhere Castaneda was cited in authoritative texts on religion, mysticism, anthropology, sociology and magic, and his work was used, among other things, as a framework for sociological analysis (Silverman, 1975). Three subsequent books by Castaneda (1973, 1975, 1976) elaborated further on the progress of his apprenticeship and were adopted as textbooks on anthropology in several US universities. Further books followed (1978, 1982, 1984, 1988), but by then doubt had descended on the whole Castaneda legend (De Mille, 1978, 1980), so much so that the last two books were described in some editions as novels, and the authenticity of the works still remains in question.

However, even allowing for the possibility that they are largely fictitious, they are nevertheless a remarkable, and apparently accurate account of the development of magical consciousness (compare for example, Chevalier, 1976). Drury (1991, p. 87) concludes that what emerges from the debate over Castaneda 'is that Carlos himself is probably the actual visionary and many of the shamanic perspectives have been implanted in the personage of the real, partially real, or unreal being known as Don Juan. In this sense it hardly matters to the person interested in states of consciousness and perception whether Don Juan is real or not since the fiction, if it is that, is authentic enough'. What is beyond doubt is the fascination they hold for the millions of readers throughout the world who have found them meaningful, and their impact on Western audiences, which has been considerable.

Drury (1978) identifies parallels between Don Juan's system, as expounded by Castaneda, and other systems of magic outside Mexico and Central America. In particular he draws attention to the similarities in the magical view of Don Juan with that found in contemporary Western magic, notably Kabbalism (an esoteric system of Judaic origin designed to induce a dramatic transformation of consciousness, and which may be viewed as the Judaic version of Taoism and Zen). It entails a structured sequence of successive imaginative experiences leading to increasingly radical modifications of consciousness and cognition, which has been likened to a kind of symbolic death and rebirth into a dimension of all-encompassing unity and harmony (Baigent, Leigh and Lincoln, 1982).

It is not necessary, however, to understand the complexities of Kabbalism, nor the details of Mexican sorcery, to see parallels between the Yaqui way of knowledge as depicted by Castaneda and other esoteric traditions. Several familiar themes emerge from Don Juan's system, the object of which is to 'stop the world' of conventional reality and see the world as it really is. He contended that the ordinary world, although generally believed to be unique and absolute, is only one of a cluster of consecutive worlds, and that man, although conditioned to perceive solely this world, still has the capability of entering into other realms 'as real, unique, absolute and engulfing' as his own world (Castaneda, 1993, p. viii). The entire teaching is concerned with acquisition of this visionary consciousness through the cultivation of intuition or inner knowledge rather than the rational mind or intellect. As in Indian teaching, the intellect is represented as a trickster or illusionist which deceives man into certain ways of seeing, thinking and acting. The teaching involves the individual learning to harness the personal powers and energies necessary to perceive other realms by way of imaginative exercises, meditation, symbolic rituals and the use of certain drugs.

In his most recent book, Castaneda (1993) identifies the art of dreaming as the most important practice developed by shamans and sorcerers in ancient times for seeing and entering into realms of being ordinarily inaccessible as a consequence of our learned ways of perceiving the world. He claims that by thoroughly explaining its principles, rationales and practices, his teacher Don Juan made the ordinarily unseen world accessible to him. He indicates that dreaming is not simply having dreams, nor day dreaming, wishing or imagining but an experience of, and participation in other worlds. It 'seems to be a sensation – a process in our bodies, an awareness in our minds' (Castaneda, 1993, p. ix), and as such is akin to Jung's concept of active imagination.

However, as Castaneda claims to have discovered for himself, and makes clear to others, understanding, much less realizing this mode of consciousness presents very real difficulties for people educated in the rational, intellectual tradition of Western culture. At one level, by clearly identifying the limitations of the verbal, logical approach, his work highlights the difficulties encountered by Westerners in attempting to comprehend the esoteric traditions of other cultures. In so doing he illustrates a new ethnomethodological framework which has since been widely adopted within anthropology and helped reinstate phenomenological methods (those which concentrate on the detailed description of conscious experience without recourse to explanation) within social science research. At another level it highlights the difficulties in trying to comprehend the nature of visionary experience. As Castaneda indicates, 'Through dreaming we can perceive other worlds, which we can certainly describe, but we can't describe what makes us perceive them. Yet we can feel how dreaming opens up these other realms' (Castaneda, 1993, p. ix). His work has also stimulated a great deal of interest and research, both academic and lay, into the practices of sorcery and shamanism, and revived interest in the traditions of Native American Indians in particular.

At a more general level, it has prompted in many readers a more intense search for alternatives to the rational culture of the West. Many people find elements of visionary and mystical experience in these works and recognize in them what appear to be universal truths.

This 'counter culture', as it was termed by Roszak (1970) represents not only a defection from the 300 year old 'cult of the fact' (Hudson's (1972) label for Western culture's obsession with reason, rationality, intellect and physicality) but also a return to the visionary, mystical and spiritual sources of antiquity, and a renewed interest in the occult, supernatural, magical and esoteric. During the 1970s these influences became increasingly infused into mainstream culture, leading the prestigious American magazine *Newsweek* to run a cover feature during 1976, in which it was claimed that the cultural revolution sweeping the country was a major transformation of general consciousness in Western society. This era of social and spiritual transition subsequently came to be referred to as 'The New Age' (Spangler, 1977; Bloom, 1991).

An influential factor in the dissemination of what might be considered 'New Age consciousness' was the establishment of the Esalen Institute, California, in 1962, by Michael Murphy and Richard Price.

The Esalen Institute

Esalen's founders aimed at establishing an educational centre committed to the development of the whole person, encompassing the spiritual and intellectual. It is a place where trends in education, religion, philosophy, the humanities, arts and science could be explored, emphasizing the achievement of full human potential. To this end, exponents of many different disciplines (religious leaders, philosophers, artists, scientists and psychologists from Eastern and Western cultures) and practices (such as yoga, meditation, relaxation, hypnosis, dance, the martial arts, massage, magic, shamanism, psychotherapy and healing) were invited to exchange views in seminars, workshops and residential programmes. The first of which was offered to the general public in 1966. By the late 1960s, Esalen was offering year-round programmes that attracted vast numbers of participants, and disseminating a diversity of eclectic psychotherapeutic and quasi-therapeutic techniques which resulted from the 'cross-fertilisation' of ideas and practices from different cultures and traditions. It became the prototype for many centres that subsequently flourished throughout the USA and Europe.

Given the rapprochement effected by Esalen it was inevitable that imaginative methods would come to the fore. Inspired by Perls, who lived and worked at Esalen for 2 years and demonstrated imaginative methods in numerous Gestalt therapy workshops and summer schools, J.O. Stevens (1971) compiled a fascinating collection of guided imagery exercises directed at the development of self-awareness. Gunther (1979) presented a series of imaginative exercises based on traditional Hindu meditational practice. Another technique to emerge, inspired partly by Gestalt therapy and partly by Eastern meditative traditions, and used extensively in humanistic therapies, is what Singer (1975) calls the 'inside the body trip'. In this technique a person complaining of physical symptoms is encouraged to relax and imagine voyaging inside his or her body in order to become aware of particular body attitudes and gain insight into physical problems. Schutz (1967) attested to the effectiveness of this imagery, not only in developing bodily awareness but also in relieving certain psychosomatic symptoms. There was subsequently a proliferation of similar guided imagery techniques.

> These methods include taking an imaginary inventory of the body, having an imaginary dialogue with internal parts of oneself, creating and interacting with an inner advisor in one's imagery, dying in one's imagination, visualizing communication between the two hemispheres of the brain, crawling into various organs of the body for observatory or reparatory purposes, exorcising the parents from various parts of the body, and regressing into the previous life (Sheikh, Kunzendorf and Sheikh, 1989, p. 491).

Psycho-imagination therapy (Shorr, 1983) also emerged during the 1980s, having been developed some 20 years previously. This is based on the premise that 'waking imagery' enables a person to bypass or break the resistances usually present in verbal expression, enabling greater awareness of internal conflicts and the mobilization of personal resources for change. This involves a change in self-concept, which is construed as a usually negative maladaptive identity attributed to the person by significant others; re-definition of which is achieved by way of insight resulting from verbalizations of imagery.

Numerous books for the general audience were also published, many of them written by psychotherapists or psychiatrists, on 'creative visualization' (Krystal, 1982, 1990; Kubler-Ross, 1982; Gawain, 1985; Gawain and King, 1988; Hay, 1988; Glouberman, 1989; Edwards, 1991; Graham, 1992, 1995), which provided similar guided imagery exercises directed towards personal growth, psychological transformation and positive mental health.

Symbolic imagery from a wide variety of occult, mystical, magical and shamanistic sources was also incorporated into various forms of psychotherapy and self-healing approaches (Schwarz, 1978; Harner, 1988). Imaginary 'power animals', typically invoked by shamans in healing rituals, re-emerged as allies of the therapist in psychotherapy (Gallegos, 1983, 1989, 1993; Harner, 1988). Native American wisdom became de rigeur (having been all but obliterated by generations of rational New World Americans) as traditional totemic symbolism became absorbed into therapeutic approaches, and the vision quest became an accepted psychotherapeutic procedure.

Within this climate numerous self-appointed and controversial shamans (Storm, 1972; Andrews, 1981; Roth, 1990) have emerged or been identified (Jamal, 1987; Krippner, 1988; Drury, 1991) and have drawn popular attention to shamanism. Michael Harner, Visiting Professor at Columbia, Yale and the University of California at Berkeley, and Associate Professor of the New School of Social Research in New York, has helped to make the experience of shamanic reality more accessible to Westerners and taught them how to apply the healing powers of the shaman in workshops at Esalen, elsewhere in the USA and in Europe.

Courses and workshops on contemporary shamanism throughout North America, Britain and Europe are advertised in numerous 'new age' journals and magazines. Indeed as Drury (1991, p. 100) observes,

> it is always possible to find some Westerners on retreats, or engaged in personal growth workshops, who enjoy the theatre of dressing up – who believe that by donning Red Indian feather headdresses or by puffing a ceremonial pipe or burning sage, that they can take on a shamanic persona. Clearly, for modern city-bound Westerners such practices are fraught with illusion – they are ultimately artificial, focusing on the external appearance of shamanism rather than the core inner, visionary experience.

Nevertheless, he concludes that there is a basic world view that can be transported from traditional shamanism to the modern context. This is increasingly evident in the field of psychological medicine. Achterberg (1985) points out that articles in psychiatry journals frequently liken the work of psychiatrists to that of the shaman. 'Shamanic' approaches to mental health and healing are being advocated within the health care professions in Britain (Money, 1992;

Buckley, 1993) and practised in America (Harner 1990). Extensive use is being made of imagery techniques in working with the bereaved (Kubler-Ross, 1982). Increasingly it is being used in therapy with emotionally disturbed children and adolescents (Oaklander, 1978) where it is used to access their feelings and to deal with stress, abuse, phobias and depression. Roet (1988) also advocates guided imagery techniques as a means by which parents can gain insight into the normally hidden realms of their children's experiences (their fears, anxieties, needs, wishes and preoccupations) and thus monitor emotional and psychological development more sensitively. Indeed, to the extent that images facilitate exploration of a person's inner world, they can assist in the development of interpersonal empathy. McKellar (1989) therefore describes images as 'empathy bridges', and considers them of value in the treatment of both neuroses and psychoses. Given this growing recognition of their usefulness, it is becoming increasingly difficult to identify areas of psychological medicine where imaginative methods are not employed. As Sheikh, Kunzendorf and Sheikh (1989, p. 489) note,

> During the last two decades, imagery has risen from a position of near disgrace to become one of the hottest topics in clinical and experimental cognitive psychology. Experimental and clinical psychologists of varied persuasions have made imagery the subject of their inquiry, and they have produced a considerable body of literature documenting that images are indeed a powerful source.

Thus in the field of psychological medicine, at least, it is clear that imaginative methods have come full circle.

Modern developments in imaginative medicine: the emergence of psychoneuroimmunology

3

O, who can hold a fire in his hand
By thinking on the frosty caucasus?
Or cloy the hungry edge of appetite
By bare imagination of a feast?
Or wallow naked in December snow
By thinking on fantastic summer's heat?
William Shakespeare: Richard II

Within Western culture, until the seventeenth century mind, body and spirit were all interrelated. However, from the seventeenth century, as a result of Cartesian philosophy which distinguished nature into two discrete realms (mind (*res cogitans*) and matter (*res extensa*)) which were separated from each other and progressively, from the soul. Psychology and medicine became divorced from religion and from each other, and developed along different paths. However, by the middle of the nineteenth century, psychological findings were beginning to make an impact on medicine. Several factors were involved in this development, but a major influence in lowering the barriers between medicine and psychology was the discovery of the unconscious mind. The concept of unconscious mental processes entered English and German philosophy in the seventeenth century. It began to flourish in Germany during the nineteenth century, but, as Hearnshaw (1989, p. 150) indicates, 'what brought it decisively within the ambit of medicine was the arrival of Mesmerism towards the end of the eighteenth century'.

MESMERISM

Franz Anton Mesmer (1734–1815) did not discover the phenomenon which came to be named after him. The priest-doctors and shamans of primitive tribes brought about similar trance-like states to those Mesmer induced in others. There are indications that a similar practice was used by healers in ancient Egypt, Greece and Rome (Edelstein and Edelstein, 1945), and subsequently by others such as Paracelsus (Webster, 1988), and the seventeenth century Irish healer Valentine Greatraks (Inglis, 1990). Hearnshaw claims that Mesmer was distinguished from them by his formulation of scientifically testable propositions which linked the phenomena with the manifestations of 'a universally distributed and continuous fluid...of an incomparably rarefied nature', and with 'properties similar to those of a magnet'.

In fact, there was nothing original or distinctive in Mesmer's formulation. The sixth century physician Galen, whose views were still influential in eighteenth century Europe, had claimed that an invisible essential fluid filled the universe, planets and all living creatures, and that health consisted in a balance of the fluid essences of mind, body, soul and the environment. Accordingly the universe was a living organism of balancing forces, and health lay in each part adjusting to every other part so that it reserved to the fullest, the capacity to direct, control and sustain the life of the whole. Such a view, as Butler (1982) observes, was, and still is, fundamental to Western traditions of magic, and has recently been revived within Western scientific thinking (Lovelock, 1979).

Also current in Mesmer's time was the notion disseminated by Paracelsus that magnets possessed special healing properties, and with their powers of polar attraction and repulsion could be used to influence this ethereal fluid. Healing by stroking and touch was also common during this period.

Mesmer simply combined these three principles, viewing the body as a magnet and illness as faulty distribution of magnetic fluid, which he attempted to redistribute by passing his hands over the body in much the way that a metal is magnetized. He believed that in this way he could realign the magnetic field associated with a sick person and effect a cure. As he was able to demonstrate striking cures, his concepts of animal magnetism and magnetic treatment, which came to be known as Mesmerism, became very popular, especially among the poor who could not afford orthodox medical treatment. In France, where Mesmer was practising, this lead to an investigation of Mesmerism by a Royal Commission, led by the US Commissioner to France, Benjamin Franklin.

Mesmer's claims for magnetic effects were systematically tested using magnetometers, which failed to detect any magnetism. The Franklin Commission reported in 1784 that there was no substance to Mesmer's claims, and that all the effects attributed to magnetism were the result only of the patient's imagination. By dismissing animal magnetism in this way the commissioners implied that Mesmeric procedures had no validity. What they failed to do was to distinguish between the procedures, which clearly did have therapeutic value and Mesmer's explanation of how they worked. They also failed to recognize that their conclusions as to how the procedures achieved their effects raised important questions about the therapeutic possibilities of the imagination. However, the Franklin report dismissed imagination along with Mesmerism. It was some 200 years later before the importance and implications of the commission's conclusions were recognized and given serious consideration.

The Franklin report discredited Mesmer, who retired into obscurity, but interest in Mesmerism and its practice continued. Dugald Stewart (1753–1828), professor of moral philosophy at Edinburgh University, was the first to recognize its scientific potential. He claimed the phenomena produced by Mesmer as 'inestimable data for extending our knowledge of the laws which regulate the connection between the human mind and our bodily organization' (Hearnshaw, 1989, p. 152). Following a demonstration of Mesmerism by Charles Lafontaine in 1841, a Scottish physician, James Braid (1795–1860) commenced a series of experiments which led him to reject Mesmer's theories and to develop new concepts and methods. In a book of 1843 he proposed that the combined state of physical relaxation and altered awareness entered into by persons who were mesmerized should be called hypnosis, from the Greek *hypnos* meaning sleep.

HYPNOSIS

By this time the rapprochement between medicine and psychology had been furthered by the Edinburgh physician John Abercrombie. In 1830, he noted that in madness, fever and other abnormal states the mind betrays capacities and extensive systems of knowledge of which it is at other times wholly unconscious. He claimed this was evidence of the existence of an unconscious region of the mind. However it was by way of hypnosis that the influence of unconscious factors on behaviour became clearly demonstrated. As a result the doctrine of the unconscious mind ceased merely to be a philosophical abstraction.

Hypnosis proved to be of great interest to both physicians and psychologists. Before the introduction of ether and chloroform, which were easier to administer and less time-consuming, it was used as the sole anaesthetic in a great number of painless operations by a number of surgeons in Britain and elsewhere. In continental Europe Liebeault (1823–1904) effected many remarkable cures with hypnosis. J.M. Charcot (1835–1893), a neurologist at the Salpêtrière mental hospital in France, demonstrated that paralysis and anaesthesia could be produced and abolished by hypnosis. The psychiatrist Paul Janet (1859–1947) used hypnosis in the exploration of multiple personality. In so doing he anticipated by several years both the importance of unconscious processes in mental illness, and the means of accessing them in psychotherapy, which subsequently were the focus of Freud's theorizing and practice. Although, as Hearnshaw points out, it was undoubtedly Freud who finally and irrevocably threw medicine and psychology together:

the striking manifestations of hypnosis brought to public attention by Mesmer towards the end of the eighteenth century and studied intensively during the early half of the nineteenth, together made it hard to deny that the mind also had an influence on the functions of the body. It seemed increasingly clear that mind and body were part of a single system. Later, in the 1920s and 1930s, the term psychosomatic was introduced to express this unity (Hearnshaw, 1989, p. 120).

A report by the British Medical Association in 1893 stated that 'as a therapeutic agent hypnosis is frequently effective in relieving pain, procuring sleep and alleviating many functional ailments', and a wealth of research worldwide has since supported these claims. The literature on the uses of hypnosis in psychotherapy and psychosomatic medicine is vast. Some idea of its scope can be gleaned from the papers presented at one European conference which report on the application of hypnosis to problems including anxiety, depression, neurological disease, trauma, obstetrics, gynaecology, smoking, drug dependency, psychoticism, asthma, malignant disease, bulimia and eating disorders, sexual deviance, impotence, phobias, aphasia, hypertension, memory loss, child abuse and multiple personality.

Among the most widely reported and demonstrated effects of hypnosis is analgesia. It has proved to be a very potent pain-killer, of value in terminal illness and childbirth (Moon and Moon, 1984). Studies have found that hypnosis is better than acupuncture, Valium, aspirin and placebos in the relief of experimentally induced pain, and that its effects are more or less equivalent with those of morphine (Stern *et al.*, 1977). Hypnosis has therefore been used to control pain (Erickson, 1959; Hilgard and le Baron, 1984), anxiety and insomnia associated with cancer (Hilgard and Hilgard, 1975; Sacerdote, 1982) and dentistry (Kent, 1986); and has been found to restore self-control lost during the course of invasive cancer treatment (Zeltzer, 1980). It has also been used to overcome anticipatory emesis and nausea associated with cancer chemotherapy, which is commonly resistant to anti-emetic drugs (Redd, Andersen and Minagawa, 1982). Its role in the improvement of immune functions has also been demonstrated (Hall, 1985).

Nevertheless, despite incontrovertible evidence of its therapeutic effects, a good deal of suspicion about hypnosis remains in both psychology and medicine. Many doctors and psychologists regard it as unscientific and mysterious. This is largely because research has failed to find a single explanation for its effects. As Wagstaff (1986) suggests, the various phenomena may require different explanations, with a range of processes interacting to give rise to effects which may vary from situation to situation and person to person. Also the explanation offered by the Franklin Commission (that imagination is solely responsible for observed effects) is generally regarded as insufficient to account for phenomena that are widely and erroneously regarded as highly unusual and otherwise impossible to achieve.

In fact there is abundant evidence that so-called hypnotic behaviour is not as remarkable as is commonly supposed, and that the feats performed under hypnosis are achievable under normal conditions (Spanos, 1986). Nevertheless the supposed discrepancy between 'normal' and hypnotic behaviour has led a number of theorists to explain the latter in terms of unusual psychological and physiological mechanisms (Orne, 1959; Sarbin, 1962; Chertok, 1969, 1981; Ellenberger, 1970). This view is challenged by other theorists who consider that well-established psychological and social processes can account for the effects very adequately (Barber, 1969, 1978; Barber, Spanos and Chaves, 1974; Wagstaff, 1981; Spanos, 1982; Naish, 1986; Bertrand and Spanos, 1989). These different assumptions are the basis of much continuing debate in what remains a highly controversial field of research. What is not contested, however, is the importance of imagery in hypnosis.

> Hypnotic suggestions do not ask subjects explicitly to enact overt behaviours, rather they inform subjects that a specific behavioural event will occur, while inviting them to engage in imaginings that are consistent with the occurrence of the behaviour...For instance, imagine a force attracting your hands toward each other...As you think of this force pulling your hands together, they will move together (Bertrand and Spanos, 1989, p. 240).

These suggestions may be augmented by imagery. Thus, for example, arm levitation, where a subject is instructed that one arm will rise higher and higher (which is a common index of a subject's suggestibility) may be accompanied by appropriate imagery, such as balloons or strings attached to the subject's hands, tugging upwards and drawing the fingers up with them.

Hence Barber (1961) attributes the effects of hypnosis to the vividness of the imagery created by the subject in response to suggestion. Certainly many nineteenth century commentators, including Alexandre Bertrand (1823), considered that hypnosis and its effects were brought about by the subject's imagination. Liebeault concurred with this view, claiming that hypnosis was brought about by auto-suggestion.

AUTO-SUGGESTION AND COUÉISM

As a chemist, Emile Coué (1857–1926) was interested in whether the imagination could perform the same function as a drug. Having experimented with auto-suggestion, he became convinced that it could. He developed it into a form of self-healing or psychotherapy which became known as Couéism, and for which he claimed a 97% success rate in overcoming his patients' presenting problems. This method of treatment became extremely popular prior to World War I, when an estimated 40 000 people were treated annually by Coué (Blythe, 1979). However, its very simplicity, comprising as it did the mental rehearsal of a series of suggestions intended to promote psychological and physical well-being, led to its falling into disrepute. Practitioners of Couésim simply repeated relevant formulae and ignored the preparatory stages of the process, such as relaxation, the resolution of unconscious conflicts, and subsequent vivid imaging of the desired outcome. Indeed, Couéism came to be seen as the mobilization of will-power, despite Coué's claims that it is not the will, but the imagination, which is of crucial importance in bringing about physiological effects.

AUTOGENIC TRAINING

The principle of auto-suggestion was taken further in autogenic training, 'a psychophysiologic form of psychotherapy which the patient carries out himself by using passive concentration upon certain combinations of psychophysiologically adapted stimuli' (Luthe, 1969, p. 309). In contrast to most forms of psychotherapy, autogenic training is directed to mental and bodily functions simultaneously. It was developed in the 1930s by the German neurologist and psychiatrist, Johannes Schultz. He described it as a 'method of rational physiological exercises designed to produce a general psychobiologic reorganization in the subject which enables him to manifest all the phenomena otherwise obtainable through hypnosis' (Schultz, 1932).

Schultz based his system on the work of the distinguished brain physiologist Oskar Vogt who, in his research into sleep and hypnosis between 1890 and 1900, found that some people are able to put themselves into a state resembling hypnosis for predetermined periods. He observed that those persons who achieved what he termed 'auto-hypnosis' had a substantial reduction of fatigue and tension, and a decrease in the incidence and severity of psychosomatic disorders, such as headache. Drawing on these observations, Schultz combined the concept of auto-hypnosis with a number of exercises designed to improve and integrate mental and physical functioning and eliminate maladjusted behaviour and its manifestations in neurotic and psychosomatic symptoms.

He noted that hypnotized subjects generally reported two characteristic sensations, a pleasurable feeling of warmth in the limbs and torso, and heaviness. Both are in fact psychological correlates of relaxation, the subjective sensation of warmth being the psychological perception of vasodilation in the peripheral arteries, and the sensation of heaviness being the perception of muscular relaxation. Schultz concluded that if he could design exercises which would enable subjects to induce these sensations in themselves he might be able to teach them to achieve the 'passive concentration' characteristic of hypnosis. He thought that once they were able to achieve this easily and rapidly it might be possible for them to progress to subtle psychological effects and to achieve a marked degree of autonomy over bodily functions. Luthe (1969) describes passive concentration as a casual attitude toward the intended outcome of concentrated activity, thereby distinguishing it from active concentration which is characterized by concern, interest, attention and goal-directed efforts regarding its outcome and functional result. Pelletier (1978, pp. 230–1) suggests that during passive concentration subjects 'learn to abandon themselves to an ongoing organismic process rather than exercising conscious will', and in so doing achieve a state of mind and body similar to the low arousal state of meditation which allows the body to self-regulate toward a more harmonious state.

Indeed in Schultz' system, as in meditation, it is necessary to minimize external stimulation and turn attention inwards. To this end there must be monotonous input to various sensory receptors and concentrated attention towards somatic processes. This is achieved primarily by mental repetition of psychophysiologically adapted suggestions, while focusing attention on the parts of the body referred to in these formulae. As such it is similar to mantra yoga and meditation, which Day (1953, p. 25) indicates has an affinity with Couéism inasmuch as it deals with positive affirmations. Furthermore Schultz claimed that given these conditions dissolution of ego boundaries occurs, as it does in yoga, producing a dream-like state of consciousness and plasticity of imagery. Like yoga it commences with physiologically oriented exercises, progressing to exercises which focus primarily on mental imagery, and finally to special exercises developed for the normalization of certain functional and organic disorders. With regular practice these lead ultimately to the self-regulation of numerous mental and physical functions. There is thus a step-wise progression through physical relaxation and mental imagery, to self-healing.

Most of the advanced stages of autogenic training involve 'the summoning and holding of certain images in the mind for examination and exploration of their effects on consciousness' (Pelletier, p. 244). Indeed they are intended to produce an intensification of psychic experience by increasing a person's ability to experience inner psychological phenomena visually (Gorton, 1959). This process commences with the rotation of the eyeballs upward and inward so that they look towards the centre of the forehead. This procedure is often recommended in other mystical and meditative practices and in hypnosis, and has been shown to induce an increase in the production of alpha rhythms of the brain (Kamiya, 1969) or to deepen a hypnotic, trance-like state of consciousness. Once this is achieved the person progresses to various exercises in which vivid colour imagery is produced. Initially holding a static, uniform colour in the mind's eye, then imagining various colour formations such as clouds, shadows or movements, then multicoloured patterns and forms, and eventually objects, such as faces, masks, statuettes and the like. The person then progresses to transforming abstract concepts such as justice, freedom and happiness into images, and elaborating fantasies pertaining to them. Eventually over a period of weeks the person progresses to images such as standing on top of a mountain or the moon, flying over clouds or seeing a sunrise, in which archetypal figures and religious themes often emerge.

At this point the individual may become an active participant in the material which comes to him and experience himself as an actor in the tableau which his mind presents...The quality of the state the trainee achieves is very like that of dreaming and is at least equally vivid and real. He begins to experience the collective dimensions or the transpersonal dimensions of consciousness. When the mind calls up scenes in which the individual begins to see himself as an active participant, the exercises are called 'film strips'. Later, when there are prolonged periods of self-participation, the visualization is called 'multi-chromatic cinerama'. In this last, most elaborate phase, where fantasy and reality alternate in the subject matter of what is 'seen', both therapist and patient may derive significant insight into the patient's unconscious. Such insights can be of great use in resolving both psychological and physiological states of disorder and psychosomatic stress (Pelletier, 1978, p. 248).

Finally, the individual progresses to imagining other persons, the aim being to provide insight into affective relationships and to promote changes in the individual's perceptions of significant others. Schultz suggested that the advanced visualization exercises of autogenic training can be employed effectively in psychotherapy, and also applied as 'Nirvana therapy' in clinically hopeless cases or in monotonous or desperate situations.

Schultz employed his system to treat both psychological and physical conditions, including peptic ulcers, indigestion, circulatory problems, angina, heart arrhythmias, obsessive behaviours, phobias, sexual problems, diabetes, asthma, migraine and allergies; and claimed a considerable degree of success. He reported that after training, subjects could modify pain thresholds in different parts of the body, block the pain of dental drilling, warm their feet by raising foot temperature as much as $3°F$, and that hypertensive patients could achieve decreases in blood pressure of 10–20%.

Autogenic training has been subjected to considerable experimental research and the impressive claims made for it by Schultz have found much support. It would appear that in the autogenic state, subjects are capable of regulating a wide range of physiological functions by way of auto-suggestion. Numerous studies cited by Luthe (1969) have reported significant physiological effects including reductions by as much as 10%, in respiratory rate, blood pressure and heart rate. Luthe (1969) reports a number of studies (Schultz, 1932; Siebenthal, 1952; Wittstock, 1956; Eiff and Jorgens, 1961) in which a significant decrease of muscle potentials was recorded during passive concentration on heaviness, and a significant reduction in patella response (Schultz, 1932; Schultz and Luthe, 1961). He also indicates that changes in peripheral circulation during passive concentration have been verified by a number of independent researchers including Binswanger (1929) and Stovkis, Renes and Landemann (1961). Extensive studies by Polzien (1961a,b,c) confirm the earlier findings of Siebenthal (1952) and Muller-Hegeman and Kohler (1961) which found a rise of skin temperature, more pronounced in distal parts of extremities than in more proximal areas, and an increase of weight in both arms during passive concentration. Changes in blood sugar level during concentration on warmth in the liver area have also been demonstrated (Marchand, 1956, 1961) as have changes in heart rate during autogenic training (Schultz and Luthe, 1959). Changes in the shape of the eyeballs and improved distance vision have been found in near-sighted people (Kelly, 1961). Autogenic training has also eliminated stomach contractions resulting from great hunger (Lewis and Sarbin, 1943) and anaesthetized against third degree burns (Gorton, 1959).

Autogenic training is used as a standard pre-operative procedure in Germany and is widely used throughout Europe, where it is integrated into the medical training programmes of many universities. It is also now used in Canada, the USA and Japan. Until recently it has been little known or practised in Britain. However, the situation is changing as a result of research, such as that of Medik and Fursland (1984) which found that 82% of all patients referred for autogenic training with a wide range of problems found it generally helpful, 74% found that it also helped specific symptoms, and most reported feeling more relaxed and confident. Horn (1986) has also reported a study of 100 healthy persons aged between 25 and 60, half of whom were allocated to physical exercise and half to autogenic training following physical and physiological tests designed to select stress variables and heart risk factors. After 2 months both groups had experienced considerable reductions in anxiety and depression, improved their scores on general health questionnaires, reported an enhanced sense of well-being, improved sleep, reduced physical tension, and showed significant reductions in resting pulse rate, blood pressure and blood fatty acids. In every respect, autogenic training proved to be as useful as exercise, which is an important finding given the results of a study (Prosser, Carson and Phillips, 1985) which demonstrated that only 14 of 215 patients having suffered heart attack were prepared to continue exercise therapy. Almost half of the patients reported finding exercise inconvenient; 30% found it boring; 25% disliked exercise without medical supervision; and a further 35% gave medical reasons for discontinuing the exercise programme. The advantage of autogenic training over exercise is that, being essentially sedentary, it can be practised by anyone, whether confined to bed or a wheelchair, and can be successfully used in work or leisure contexts. Moreover, once mastered it is the fastest method of achieving passive concentration. Unlike yoga, it does not take much time. Another advantage emphasised by Wilson (1987) is that the body is not expected to react in a stereotyped way. Apart from the increasing speed of reaction to suggestions, subtle changes constantly take place as the intensity of the practice grows and the suggestions can be changed to suit current needs as well as distant aims.

Luthe therefore concludes that 'both clinical results and experimental data indicate that autogenic training operates in a highly differentiated field of bodily self-regulation and that with the help of autogenic principles it is possible to use one's brain to influence certain bodily and mental functions effectively' (Luthe, 1969, p. 317).

POSITIVE THINKING AND IMAGERY

Recognition of the power of suggestion in self-regulation is defined by Stoyva (1976, p. 2) as 'the endeavour to modify voluntarily one's own physiological activity, behavior, or process of consciousness'. It has led many therapists to encourage auto-suggestion, now more commonly referred to as 'positive thinking', in their patients (Roet, 1987; Manning, 1989), and books on the subject (Jampolsky, 1979) have become best-sellers. However, as Singer (1975, p. 224) points out:

> The power of positive imagery, as one might call this technique, should not be taken lightly. It is not the same as simply saying nice things to oneself or pepping oneself up, as encouraged in a number of popular self-help books on mental health...It involves, first of all, relaxing the patient and encouraging him to generate very vivid scenes that are associated in his mind with very specific positive emotions such as joy and peacefulness...The extensive relaxation plus fixation on these positive images can create a state of private peacefulness that often will help counteract the anxiety aroused by the thought of various phobic events...Extensions of the positive imagery method also provide opportunities for patients to learn how to distract themselves from the kind of recurring attention to a painful or frightening situation that reinforces its negative content. Part of treatment may include training people to develop a repertory of positive images to draw on during periods of excessive stress.

AUTONOMIC SELF-REGULATION

The self-regulation of physiological functions was further emphasized in research instigated by I.P. Pavlov (1849–1936), the Russian physiologist who was awarded the Nobel prize for his work on gastric secretions. In the course of an experimental programme, Pavlov noted that these secretions could be produced by 'psychic' causes, and that dogs could be conditioned to salivate to the sound of a bell by pairing it with a food stimulus. Further investigations revealed that by rewarding desired performance in this way dogs could learn to effect other physiological functions ordinarily considered to be autonomic or involuntary, to the extent of changing their body temperature by controlling blood flow to one leg at a time. Pavlov considered these conditioned reflexes, as he termed them, to be the result of unconscious learning processes which could be studied objectively, and he proceeded to do so for over 30 years. In so doing he discovered a number of significant factors about the mechanisms involved in behavioural processes and exerted a profound effect on the subsequent development of the behaviourist movement and on various learning theories which dominated American psychology for the next quarter of a century.

Influenced by Pavlov's work on conditioned reflexes, behaviourists confined themselves to studying the effects of unconscious learning on bodily responses, chiefly in rats. Their research showed that, by rewarding desired performance rats could be trained to salivate, accelerate or slow their heart rate and alter blood pressure, control circulation in the stomach wall, and direct heat to one or other ear. One celebrated rat even learned to fire an individual nerve cell (Miller, 1969). Subsequently, they asserted that unconscious learning applied to all animal and human responses (Watson, 1916, 1925), including vasodilation and constriction (Menzies, 1937, 1941), heart rate acceleration and deceleration (Wegner and Zeaman, 1958; Furedy and Poulos, 1976); immuno-suppression and immuno-enhancement (Ader, 1985).

However, as Norris (1989) indicates, Indian masters of yoga have taught their students to self-regulate their psychological and psychophysiological processes consciously and voluntarily for over 5000 years, and for centuries many other people around the world have used various aspects of self-regulation, particularly in healing rituals. Until relatively recently, in the West, this voluntary control of biological processes was generally associated with paranormal capacities or dismissed as fanciful. However, from the 1930s onwards a number of studies indicated that so called autonomic functions could be brought under voluntary control by human subjects during meditation.

MEDITATION

In 1935 the French cardiologist, Thérèse Brosse, recorded measures of heart rate control in Indian yogis during meditation indicative of an advanced voluntary capacity to regulate autonomic functions including metabolic rate. Subsequently Sugi and Akutsu (1964) found that during meditation the oxygen consumption of Zen monks decreased by 20%, and their carbon dioxide output also decreased, indicating a slowing of metabolism. Anand, Chhina and Singh (1961a) reported a similar finding in their study of an Indian yogi, Swami Ramananda. Such studies strongly suggested that advanced meditators could produce these effects through control of the autonomic nervous system during meditation. This was confirmed by investigations conducted within the Voluntary Controls Program at the Menninger Foundation of the yogi, Swami Rama. He demonstrated his ability to stop his heart from pumping blood by putting it into 'atrial flutter', and afterwards gave a lecture on how this feat was achieved. In another demonstration, he controlled vascular behaviour in two areas of his hand less than two inches apart, making one area hotter and the other simultaneously colder, and producing a temperature difference of 10°F without at any time moving his hands (Green and Green, 1977). Voluntary control of the autonomic nervous system, and control of pain, bleeding and healing was also demonstrated in the laboratories of the Menninger Foundation. It was also demonstrated at the Langley Porter Neuropsychiatric Institute by

Jack Schwarz, who inserted a large diameter, unsterilized knitting needle completely through his left bicep without any change in his recorded heart rate or skin temperature, or indicating stress of any kind. He too was able to explain how this was possible, insisting that 'the abilities that I demonstrated in these experiments are within everyone's reach, and achievable by way of creative meditation' (Schwarz, 1978, p. 11).

During the 1950s and 1960s, research was facilitated by the development of sophisticated recording devices, notably the electroencephalogram which detects the electrical rhythms generated by the brain. Explorations with this apparatus showed that meditation produces changes in brain wave activity (Karamatsu and Hirai, 1966, 1969; Benson and Zlipper, 1975; Hirai, 1975). During meditation, yogis demonstrated brain wave activity characteristic of deep relaxation with eyes closed, and were not distracted by external stimuli such as strong light, loud noises, being burned with hot glass tubing, or vibrations from a tuning fork. This suggests an association between brain wave regulation and the ability to establish autonomic control. They also found that when practising meditation yogis showed an increased pain threshold to cold water and could keep a hand in water at 4°C for 45–55 minutes without experiencing discomfort (Anand, Chhina and Singh, 1961b).

Research also established that during meditation skin resistance to an electric current increases, indicating greater relaxation of the subjects. The pattern of physiological alteration occurring during meditation is characterized by: an extreme slowing of respiration to between four and six breaths per minute; a more than 70% increase in the electrical resistance of the skin; a predominance of alpha wave activity in the brain; and a slowing of the heart rate from 72 to 24 beats per minute, which is suggestive of a state of deep relaxation (Bagchi and Wenger, 1959). Indeed numerous studies indicate that meditation is more refreshing than sleep (Wallace, 1970), and that after commencing regular meditation subjects require less sleep than formerly (Bloomfield, Cain and Jaffe, 1975).

Various psychological effects were also claimed for meditators including: greater psychological stability (Schwartz and Goleman, 1976); greater autonomic stability (Orme-Johnson, 1973); lower anxiety (Linden, 1973; Nidich, Seaman and Dreskin, 1973); internal locus of control and a sense of being effective in the world rather than a passive victim of circumstance (Schwartz and Goleman, 1976). All of which are essential goals of psychotherapy and psychosomatic medicine. A substantial reduction in headaches, colds, insomnia, and the use of alcohol, cigarettes and coffee, has been found among meditators, and dietary changes such as eating less meat. Meditators also report more positive mood states, regular daily routines, and a lower incidence of somatic complaints (Schwartz, 1973). Meditation has also proved successful in the treatment of asthma (Honsberger and Wilson, 1973), hypertension (Wallace and Benson, 1972; Benson et al., 1974; Cooper and Aygen, 1978) and phobias (Boudreau, 1972).

Yoga has also been shown to have positive therapeutic benefits in the treatment of both psychosomatic and organic disorders, notably in the management of hypertension (Patel, 1973; Patel and Datey, 1975; Dostalek, 1987), where it has been shown to have beneficial effects similar to the tranquillizer diazepam. It has also proved effective in the treatment of venous and lymphatic insufficiency, peripheral artery disease, chronic bronchitis, emphysema and sinusitis (Monjo, 1987).

During the 1970s, a great deal of research was conducted on transcendental meditation which had recently been introduced to the West by Maharishi Mahesh Yogi. It was studied, not only because it was practised by millions of his followers, but also because its well-standardized procedures enabled large-scale studies to be conducted under reasonably well-controlled conditions. This research confirmed earlier findings that during meditation there is a reduction in metabolic rate indicated by: a decreased rate and volume of respiration, decreased elimination of carbon dioxide; low level of arterial blood pressure; decline in blood lactate level; increase in skin resistance; slowing of heart rate; and intensification of alpha waves in the brain (Wallace and Benson, 1972; Benson and Zlipper, 1975).

BIOFEEDBACK

In response to these studies of voluntary autonomic regulation, behaviourists attempted to account for autonomic training 'scientifically': that is, without recourse to mental explanations. In 1969, the term 'biofeedback' was first used to describe investigations into voluntary control of various internal processes. Biofeedback is based on the premise that if an individual can become aware of some bodily function of which he is normally unaware, he can become able to control it, and this awareness can be achieved by providing some feedback about that function. Gradually it emerged that any neurophysiological or other biological function that can be monitored or amplified and feedback can be regulated. It has been established that over a period of weeks subjects can: acquire control of their heartbeat (Hnatiow and Lang, 1965; Lang, 1967); overcome rhythmic disabilities of atrial fibrillation and premature ventricular contraction (Engel, 1972); control high blood pressure without the use of drugs (Elder, 1977); vary the temperature of their hands (Green, 1969); control brain waves (Kamiya, 1968); and regulate stomach acidity (Gorman and Kamiya, 1972). By 1972, Ornstein was able to observe that, whereas a few years previously it would have been considered 'paranormal' to claim control over blood pressure, it was now possible for a subject in a psychological experiment to learn some measure of blood pressure control in half an hour.

Biofeedback has been employed successfully in the treatment of migraine and tension headache (where it has been demonstrated to be more effective than diazepam) (Paiva et al., 1982) and in ulcerative colitis and spastic colon. Pelletier (1978) reports that it has been used to: help patients regain control after periods of dysporesis; teach individuals bronchial tube diameter, which has implications for the control of asthma and other respiratory disease; assist in regulation of chronic diarrhoea and constipation; and to retrain patients with faecal incontinence resulting from organic impairment. He also reports encouraging results in: treating hemiplegic patients paralysed for over 6 months (Johnson and Gorton, 1973); in partial paralysis resulting from stroke, Bell's palsy and other muscular problems (Marinacci, 1968); retraining severed facial nerves (Booker, Rubow and Coleman, 1969); and various cardiovascular disorders (Brener and Kleinman, 1970). Success in improving immune functions with biofeedback has also been reported by Peavey (1982).

Norris (1989) indicates that biofeedback has also been used successfully and routinely in the treatment of tension and migraine headache, angina pectoris, painful menstruation, sacroiliac pain, neurodermatitis, rheumatoid arthritis, asthma, tachycardia, arrhythmia, gastric and duodenal ulcer, cardiospasm, pylorospasm, nausea and vomiting, regional enteritis, ulcerative colitis and frequency of micturition. Disorders of the circulatory system, including Raynaud's disease, Burger's disease, intermittent claudication, other peripheral vascular disorders and circulatory complications accompanying diabetes and other illnesses, can be controlled and eliminated with self-regulation. Anxiety disorders, including panic disorders and phobias, can also be treated effectively with biofeedback. She concludes:

> We have long known that the muscles of the heart, stomach, and intestines have responded to images and emotions; thinking of something frightful leads to fear, which leads to vascular and intestinal responses. Biofeedback is showing that these same 'involuntary' muscles also respond to volition and visualization. Biofeedback is making this knowledge and these abilities accessible to everyone, and biofeedback is making our potential for conscious control of the unconscious scientific, measurable, and verifiable (Norris, 1989, p. 279).

Biofeedback has not only demonstrated that conscious control of bodily processes is possible but it has also focused attention on the role of imagery in such self-regulation. Pavlov found that not all subjects can be successfully conditioned, attributing unsuccessful conditioning to innate physiological inhibition in the subjects. However, studies have linked the variability of conditioning in human subjects to differences in imaging. Indeed Achterberg (1985) indicates that poor imagers who are unable to fantasize and who seldom remember dreams have most difficulty in achieving the biofeedback response. Certainly Mangan (1974) found that the strength of appetitive galvanic skin response conditioning was positively correlated with the vividness of subjects' tactile imagery. Similarly Arabian and Furedy (1983) found that heart rate deceleration conditioning is stronger in a group of vivid imagers than in a group of poor imagers. On this basis Sheikh et al. (1989) claim that the Pavlovian conditioning of autonomic responses is mediated by mental imagery.

Others attribute individual differences in the effectiveness of biofeedback to individual differences in imaging ability, indicating that subjects who produce more vivid imagery have been found to produce greater heart rate increases (Hirschman and Favaro, 1986), greater electrodermal activity (Ikeda and Hirai, 1976), and greater electrodermal control (Kunzendorf and Bradbury, 1983). They also observe that the effectiveness of biofeedback has been linked not only to the ability to image but also to the use of imagery during biofeedback. Roberts, Kewman and MacDonald (1973) found that subjects who successfully altered local skin temperature were those who spontaneously imagined such temperature alteration. Similarly subjects who successfully lowered and raised blood pressure and heart rate were those who spontaneously imagined tranquillity in association with the former and emotional agitation with the latter (Schwartz, 1975; Bell and Schwartz, 1975; White, Holmes and Bennett, 1977; Takahashi, 1984). Other studies (LeBouef and Wilson, 1978; Qualls and Sheehan, 1979) have shown that during biofeedback for relaxation, subjects who successfully attenuated their electromyographic responses were those who spontaneously imagined tranquillity.

Research has explicitly compared the effectiveness of biofeedback alone, biofeedback with imagining instructions and imaging without feedback. In research on vasomotor control (Herzfeld and Taub, 1980; Okhuma, 1985) it has been found that biofeedback with instructions to imagine warmth, produces greater skin temperature increases than biofeedback alone. In research on relaxation, biofeedback augmented by imagery has been found to produce greater electromyographic decrements than biofeedback alone (Qualls and Sheehan, 1981a). However, as Sheikh, Kunzendorf and Sheikh (1989) indicate, for some subjects biofeedback interfered with imagery (Qualls and Sheehan, 1981a,b). In a study of heart rate control by Shea (1985), smaller heart rate changes were produced by biofeedback than by emotional imaging without biofeedback and by hypnotic suggestion without biofeedback. They conclude, therefore:

Collectively, the above studies suggest that many successful effects of biofeedback can be reduced to autonomic effects of mental imaging. Moreover, the last study raises the possibility that many autonomic effects of hypnotic suggestion also can be reduced to effects of mental imaging (Sheikh, Kunzendorf and Sheikh, 1989, p. 496).

This conclusion is further supported by modern understanding of the placebo effect.

PLACEBO EFFECT

As noted in Chapter 1, the French essayist Montaigne anticipated modern understanding of the placebo effect by some 400 years, indicating that the imagination had power to cure as well as to kill. A dramatic contemporary example of this is provided by Siegel (1990, p. 96), who relates the story of the cardiologist Bernard Lown who was

> on his rounds with his students when he pointed out a critically ill patient who had what he called 'a wholesome, very good third-sound gallop' to his heart. In medical terminology a gallop rhythm means that the heart is badly damaged and dilated. There was nothing further to be done for this man, and little hope for his recovery. None the less he did make an amazing return to health, and explained why some months later. As soon as he heard Dr Lown describe his heart as having a 'wholesome gallop', he said, he figured that meant it had a strong kick to it, like a horse, and he then became optimistic about his condition and knew that he would recover – which he did.

A deliberate attempt by a contemporary American doctor to alter a patient's image of his state of health is reported by Dossey (1982). He describes one of his colleagues 'pitting his medicine against that of an adversary' by conducting a 'de-hexing' ceremony, and thereby successfully curing a patient who was dying in response to a shaman's spell. Indeed, medical practitioners throughout history have quite deliberately exploited the power of the imagination in their use of placebos. These are imitation medicines or procedures with no intrinsic therapeutic value applied more to please and placate the patient (as is reflected in the origin of the term, the Latin *placebo* meaning 'I shall please') than for any organic purpose. Shapiro (1960) claims it highly probable that until relatively recently almost all medications were placebos. He notes that patients in ancient Egypt were treated with lizards' blood, crocodile dung, swine's teeth, asses' hooves, putrid meat and such like, yet there is little doubt that patients considered these treatments effective, paid highly for them, and revered their physicians.

Placebos have been demonstrated to be as, or more, effective than real medicines in the treatment of pain and a wide variety of diseases ranging from hay fever to rheumatoid arthritis (Beecher, 1955; Rossi, 1986), which implicate the autonomic, endocrine and immune systems. However, within the medical profession the placebo, or 'doctor who resides within', as Cousins (1981b) has termed it, is widely regarded as a nuisance factor that contaminates the effects of 'real' treatments. For this reason, placebos are used in control studies to determine the efficacy of medicinal drugs. 'The effect of the placebo has been well demonstrated in experimental settings, and must be 'controlled for' in all drug studies. In other words, when a drug is tested, a group of subjects are given placebos, or fakes that look like the real thing in order to find out exactly how much of the drug's effectiveness is really in the patient's imagination' (Achterberg, 1985, pp. 85–6). It is only relatively recently, therefore, that these effects have been investigated seriously. Indeed within traditional Western medicine 'placebo' is a pejorative term, with connotations of quackery and pseudomedicine. Nevertheless within medicine it is also widely acknowledged that the prescription slip, rather than what is written on it, is often the vital ingredient in recovery. As Cousins (1981a) observed, to the patient this piece of paper with its apparently unbreakable code, is often a certificate of assured recovery, the doctor's promise of restored health. Indeed the doctor is the most powerful placebo of all, in that the chances of successful treatment seem to be directly proportional to the quality of the patient–doctor relationship. In other words, to the extent that the patient imagines the doctor's interventions can and will be effective.

Wagstaff (1987) suggests that placing relaxation, imagery and suggestion techniques within the context of hypnosis or any other therapy may simply be a ritual that culminates in some patients believing that the treatments will be effective. Hypnosis may therefore be a placebo, which for some patients, in some circumstances, is highly effective. Such a view is consistent with the observation made by Bowers (1976, p. 152), that 'human suffering responds to the spoken word rendered by compassionate persons cast in the role of healer'. It is also consistent with the recently acknowledged negative placebo or nocebo effect (Siegel, 1986), whereby treatment known to be effective does not work because an individual does not expect it to (Shapiro and Morris, 1978). Rossi (1986) illustrates this phenomenon by reporting the case of a Mr Wright who achieved a remarkable remission in his cancer in response to the newly introduced and much acclaimed 'wonder drug' Krebiozen, only to succumb quickly to the disease when the drug was derided as ineffective.

It is perhaps fair, to claim that some degree of placebo reaction is involved in the administration of every medication and therapeutic procedure. Indeed, Rossi (1986) claims that studies suggest a 55% placebo response in many, if not all, healing procedures. This response is likely to vary according to the circumstances and physiological make-up of the individual (Barber, 1987). However, to claim that the effectiveness of these approaches is no more than a placebo effect is highly controversial. Nevertheless, the use of placebos in drug trials is an implicit acknowledgement of the power of the imagination, as Achterberg (1985, pp. 85–6) points out:

> The fact that the placebo effect has been identified in thousands of drug studies is stark and incontrovertible testimony to the role of the imagination in health. The wonder is that scientists have invested so much effort in 'controlling' for it, and so little in identifying how it might be used to best advantage in health care.

This point is further elaborated by Cousins (1981b, pp. 19–20):

> What is most significant about placebos is not so much the verdict they supply on the efficacy of new drugs as the clear proof that what passes through the mind can produce alterations in the body's chemistry. These facts also indicate that the same pathways and connections that come into play through the use of placebos can be activated without placebos.

This awareness underpins the newly emergent and highly interdisciplinary of psychoneuroimmunology, which attempts to explain the mechanisms by which the mind works upon the body to influence illness, health and healing.

PSYCHONEUROIMMUNOLOGY

The functions of the immune system can broadly be classified into cellular and humoral immunity. The former refers to the responses of cells that combat viral infection and bacteria and are involved in reactions against transplanted tissue and tumours. T-lymphocytes, white blood cells involved in the cellular immune response, are sub-divided into several classes on the basis of their function. They include T-helper/inducer and T/suppressor/cytoxic lymphocytes (Kennedy, Kiecolt-Glaser and Glaser, 1988). The former stimulate the production of antibody from B-lymphocytes and also several important substances called lymphokines which enhance immune response and promote the replication of T-helper cells, the functions of which are critical for the immune response and the deficiency of which can result in immunodeficiency.

T-suppressor lymphocytes down-regulate the immune response and inhibit antibody production through their influence on T-helper cells. The helper to suppressor cell ratio is sometimes used as a global index of immune function (Kennedy, Kiecolt-Glaser and Glaser, 1988), hence low helper to suppressor cell ratios are often found in AIDS patients and other populations of immuno-suppressed individuals. The relative percentages of T-helper and T-suppressor lymphocytes are measured using specific monoclonal antibodies.

In contrast to cellular immunity, humoral immunity refers to the production of antibodies by B-lymphocytes. Antibody molecules are synthesized against, and bind to, foreign proteins or antigens, foreign substances which may trigger the immune response.

During the 1920s, Pavlov established that guinea-pigs could be conditioned to produce specific antibodies in response to being handled by research workers in the laboratory. Some 50 years later a similar discovery was made during a Pavlovian learning experiment on conditioned aversion. It was found that the immune system of rats can be conditioned by experience (Ader and Cohen, 1975), and that they can learn to enhance or suppress immune functions. The finding that cells in the immune system of rodents could be trained in the same manner as Pavlov's dogs initially attracted a good deal of scepticism, but has since been demonstrated conclusively in numerous studies (Ader, 1981, 1983; Ader and Cohen, 1981; Gorczpynski, Macrae and Kennedy, 1982; Bovberg, Ader and Cohen, 1984). Research findings from hundreds of studies relating to the influence of the mind on immunity have now been published. All of them point to the conclusion that the immune system is controlled by the brain, whose structures, particularly those involved in emotion, such as the hypothalamus and pituitary gland, can be artificially stimulated to increase or decrease immune functioning (Achterberg, 1985).

The connection between the autonomic system and emotional states was first indicated by W.B. Cannon in 1929. By the 1950s it had been established that a close affinity exists between some neurotransmitters and some endocrines, and between the pituitary, or master gland, and one of the chief regulating systems of the brain, the hypothalamus (Beach, 1948; Harris, 1955). It thus became clear that hormones are a more important regulator of behaviour than had previously been suspected by most psychologists. This new awareness gave rise to a new field of investigation, that of psychoneuroendocrinology, which was the precursor of psychoneuroimmunology (Hearnshaw, 1989).

The endocrine system was thought to be the sole mediator between the brain and immune system. Then in the 1980s, neural projections were identified in both rats and mice from the spinal cord and medulla to the thymus gland, (which stimulates the production of the immune system's T-cells). This suggested a role for these structures in the regulation of thymic function. As Achterberg (1985) points out, this established the role of so-called lower brain areas with regard to immunity, but not of the mind, which is usually synonymous with the higher areas or cortex of the brain. However, the hypothalamus, which has an important regulatory role in immune function, is intimately connected to the limbic system, part of the brain involved in emotion.

The limbic system, in turn, forms a connecting network with the frontal lobes, which are the most evolved part of the cortex itself and believed to be critical for imagery and for planning the future (Achterberg, 1985, p. 167).

However the existence of connections between the brain and immune system raises the question whether actual behaviour or events known to be modulated by various brain areas can be associated with changes in immune functions, and whether the findings of animal studies can be generalized to man.

AFFECTIVE FACTORS AND ILLNESS

The influence of affect in the onset and development of human illness has long been recognized. Galen observed that cancer more commonly occurs in women of melancholic disposition than in those of sanguine personality type. This view was later supported by the surgeon Richard Guy (1759), and by many physicians throughout history, including Amussat (1854), Burrows (1783), Nunn (1822), Paget (1870) and Parker (1885). It has also been supported by modern studies which have found that certain personality traits are characteristically associated with cancer patients (Kissen and Eysenck, 1962; Kissen and Eysenck, 1963, 1964, 1967; LeShan, 1966; Solomon, 1969; Abse et al., 1974; Achterberg, Simonton and Simonton, 1977).

Other psychological factors have been identified in cancer patients, including repression and denial of emotions, inability to express hostile feelings, poor outlet for emotional discharge, a tendency toward self-sacrifice and blame, rigidity, impaired self-awareness and a predisposition to hopelessness and despair. Reich (1975) described cancer as a disease following emotional resignation and hopelessness. Manning (1988) has suggested that it occurs in those who, in trying to gain approval from others, suppress anger and other negative emotions. Research evidence strongly suggests that cancer patients characteristically suppress emotion and seem to ignore negative feelings such as hostility, depression and guilt. Benign and malignant breast cancer patients have been found to differ in their expression of anger (Greer, Morris and Pettingdale, 1979). Long-term survivors of cancer express higher levels of hostility, anxiety, alienation and other negative emotions than short-term survivors (Derogatis, Abeloff and Melisarotos, 1979). Patients with malignant tumours have also been found to be more repressed in the expression of anxiety (Temoshok and Heller, 1981) and more passive and appeasing (Temoshok, 1985). By contrast, patients who express emotion freely and show active determination to fight their disease have been found to live longer than meek, passive, compliant or defeatist types (Meares, 1977). Cancer patients also have a greater tendency to hold resentment and not forgive, self pity, a poor ability to develop and maintain long-term relationships, and poor self-image (Simonton and Simonton, 1975).

Recognition of these tendencies, together with those toward conformity and compliance, led Temoshok and Heller (1981) to propose a cancer-prone or Type C personality. Evidence in support of this has been provided by some investigators (Riley, 1981; Shekelle et al., 1981; Greer and Watson, 1985), but not others (Dattore, Schontz and Coyne, 1980), leading Schmale and Iker (1971) to argue that cancer patients are no different from patients who develop other serious illnesses. Certainly a number of studies suggest a common pattern of helplessness and hopelessness in both psychological and physical disease. Women who develop rheumatoid arthritis have been found to be tense, moody, depressed, and to show denial and inhibition in the expression of anger (Moos, 1964; Moos and Solomon, 1964a,b, 1965a,b). Affective factors have been linked with respiratory, allergic and infectious diseases (Canter, 1972; Kasl, Evans and Neiderman, 1979; Kleiger and Kinsman, 1980; Dirks, Robinson and Diirks, 1981).

Nevertheless, as Hughes (1987) indicates, there are numerous difficulties in studying possible psychological causes of any illness, especially cancer. Although spoken of as one illness, cancer takes many forms which may have quite different causes. Factors which may be responsible for the initial onset of the disease may be quite different from those involved in its subsequent development. Onset may occur many years prior to any detectable signs of the disease, and factors which are cited as antecedent conditions may have occurred after the cancer became established. Retrospective studies of cancer therefore have several pitfalls, including the likelihood that the presence of cancer, whether recognized by the patient or not, may have influenced their psychological state by its physical effects on the brain and body chemistry. Accordingly the problems involved in designing research studies which will produce valid information about psychological precursors of cancer or other diseases are formidable. Currently there is no generally accepted means of exactly defining and measuring many of the psychological variables investigated, with the result that the findings of different studies vary with the different methods employed, and are not always comparable.

However, although the link between affect and illness is weak it may indicate a consistent mechanism at work. Pert (1986, 1987) has reviewed and discussed the connections and communication system between the limbic system, neuropeptides and the immune system and concluded that these emotion-affecting neuropeptides control the migration of human monocytes in healing and disease. She has established that mood or emotionally modulated areas of the brain, the amygdala and hypothalamus, have 40 times the number of neuropeptide receptors than other areas of the brain. This suggests that these substances function in the biochemical mediation of emotion.

Pelletier and Herzing (1989) argue that the presence of neuropeptide receptors on immune cells, together with the ability of these cells to learn, recall and produce neuropeptides themselves, suggests an interactive network of information flow between the brain and immune system, a system in which direct control of emotions may have immunological consequences. As they indicate, the involvement of neuropeptides in biochemical mediation of emotion, and their possible function in communication between the brain and immune system is not a new observation, but is one that finds increasingly supportive evidence. The implications of this involvement are considerable:

> If neuropeptides mediate emotion in the limbic system, either through normal pathways or through immune-cell production, then emotional modulation, via cognitive control, may direct the movement of immune cells via the production of neuropeptides by the CNS or the immune cells themselves. This suggests that the brain can communicate through the limbic system to the immune system or that the immune system can communicate to the brain through the limbic system. In another possible scenario, the brain would have direct access to the immune system via direct CNS links, circumventing the limbic system, and vice versa. If the immune system and the nervous system are so closely linked, it is possible that mental/emotional illness may show concomitant immune system abnormalities (some evidence exists to verify this). That there are emotional as well as cognitive channels that may modulate the immune system also suggests that personality, emotional stability, and cognitive control or awareness of situational variables may have direct immunological consequences on health (Pelletier and Herzing, 1989, pp. 354–5).

Pert's findings have been interpreted as some of the best evidence for the direct, causal influence of mind and emotions on immunity, but as Pelletier and Herzing point out, other explanations have to be considered. These include genetic factors that determine brain development, cerebral laterality, personality and immunity:

> Immunity markers, such as NK cell activity, may be genetic markers for personality and affective disorders rather than caused by them. Personality or emotional states may be linked to socioeconomic factors that have demonstrable effects on higher disease rates in cancer, infections and heart disease. Finally, genetic and/or environmental factors may have an impact upon both psychological and immunological parameters resulting in a noncausal linking. A correlation seems evident, but causation remains an open issue (Pelletier and Herzing, 1989, p. 355).

However, the effects of stress on immune function seem to provide more clear cut evidence for a direct link between psychological events and immunity in both animals and humans.

STRESS

The concept of stress was not clearly formulated until 1926 when it was introduced by Hans Selye, who later defined it as 'the non-specific response of the body to any demand made upon it' (Selye, 1974). He noted that nervous and endocrine changes occurred in reaction to prolonged stress, resulting in a number of physiological effects, including the suppression of immune functions. It is clear from most clinical and experimental trials that stress results in immune suppression.

> Chronic stress may particularly result in immunosuppression by acting through the hypothalamic–pituitary–adrenal pathway. Under stress, the hypothalamus produces a corticotrophin-releasing factor that triggers the secretion of adrenocorticotropic hormone (ACTH) by the pituitary. In turn, ACTH stimulates the adrenals to secrete the corticosteroid hormones, which result in immunosuppression. In addition to the corticosteroids, the stress response also results in the production of brain chemistries (including epinephrine, endorphins, dopamine, and prostaglandins), which also suppress the cellular production of antibodies (Pelletier and Herzing, 1989, pp. 356–7).

Receptors for a variety of hormones and neurotransmitters that are produced during stress have been discovered on lymphocytes (Bishopric, Cohen and Leftowitz, 1980; Borysenko and Borysenko, 1982; Hucklebridge, 1990), and evidence for a functional link between the nervous and immune systems has been provided (Bulloch and Moore, 1981; Williams et al., 1981).

Many studies (reviewed by Palmblad (1981) and Jemmott and Locke (1984)) have linked disease with stress. Broadly the evidence suggests that when stress reactions are prolonged the primary action of the adrenal hormones is to suppress the work of the immune system. Furthermore, the massive changes sustained during prolonged stress go beyond immune activity to every gland targeted by the pituitary, and therefore influence reproduction, growth, and the integrity and well-being of the body at the cellular level (Achterberg, 1985). Thus what is in the short term an adaptive response can eventually give rise to every conceivable disease.

Other studies have linked disease with specific stress, such as that resulting from depression (Schleifer et al., 1984; Anonymous, 1987), marital disturbance (Somers, 1979; Verbrugge, 1979), and hopelessness (Goodkin, Antoni and Blaney, 1986). Research at Ohio State University College of Medicine since 1982 has been examining the effects of various life events on the immune system. Academic examinations have been found to be associated with transient immunosuppression effects in medical students (Kiecolt-Glaser et al., 1984; Glaser et al., 1985a,b). Several qualitative and quantitative changes in lymphocytes were found in association with examinations, including decreases in the percentages of T-helper lymphocytes and decreases in their ability to respond to mitogens (substances that stimulate cell proliferation and are thought to mimic naturally occurring antigens in the environment). Additionally, decreases in the number of natural killer (NK) cells were found during examinations. NK cells are thought to be involved in the surveillance and destruction of virus-infected cells and tumour cells, and therefore to have a role in anti-tumour surveillance (Herberman, 1982; Herberman et al., 1982; Kiecolt-Glaser et al., 1986). Changes in antibody levels to latent herpes viruses were also associated with examinations, suggesting virus reactivation probably as a result of poorer cellular immune system competence. Self-report data collected during and one month prior to the examinations confirmed that this period was associated with greater distress than baseline periods. Moreover, the immunological changes did not appear to be a function of nutritional status, as measured by plasma protein markers. Other investigators have also reported a relationship between academic examination stress and changes in immunity (Dorian et al., 1982; Jemmott et al., 1983); and between inhibited power motivation and immunity (McClelland et al., 1980, 1982; McClelland and Jemmott, 1980).

Kiecolt-Glaser et al. (1984) also found that lonely students showed poorer immune function than those who did not report loneliness. These findings are consistent with those of a later study (Kiecolt-Glaser et al., 1986) which revealed poorer immune responses in separated and divorced women than in married women, and suggests that satisfaction with interpersonal relationships may be related to certain aspects of immunity.

Immunological consequences have also been associated with changes in interpersonal relationships. Significant deficits in immune function have been documented in individuals following the death of a spouse (Bartrop et al., 1977; Schleifer et al., 1983). Bereaved spouses are reported to be a high risk from certain diseases and to have higher mortality rates than non-bereaved subjects (Windholz, Marmar and Horowitz, 1985). Hucklebridge (1993) notes that depressed immune function may also be associated with post-natal depression, suggesting that dysphoria or negative changes in mood correlate with reduced immune response.

He also observes that relatively minor life events may be the precursor to colds and viruses. This suggests that psychological events, such the frustration of missing a bus, may reduce the secretion of immunoglobin (IGA) across mucous surfaces. This is thought to be very important in defending the nose and gut from invading bacteria, making them more susceptible to colds and viruses.

Research on animals provides abundant support for the relationship between psychological and immunological variables reported in humans. Pelletier and Herzing (1989) indicate that stress has been found to reduce immunocompetence in humoral immunity (Edwards and Dean, 1977; Edwards et al., 1980) cellular immunity (Joasoo and Mckenzie, 1976; Reite, Harbeck and Hoffman, 1981; Laudenslager, Reite and Harbeck, 1982), and enhanced susceptibility to neoplastic disease (Riley, 1981), infectious disease (Mohamed and Hanson, 1980), and autoimmune diseases (Amkraut, Solomon and Kraemer, 1971). Stressful events such as overcrowding and exposure to high intensity sound have also been found to correlate with increased susceptibility to infections (Davis and Read, 1958; Jensen and Rasmussen, 1963; Brayton and Brain, 1975).

Stress and cancer

A good deal of research, both animal and human, has highlighted the connection between stress and cancer. There is nothing new in this idea. Timms (1989) notes that Gendron in 1701 and the surgeon Richard Guy in 1759 highlighted the possible role of adverse life events in the development of cancer. Since then others have cited loss as an antecedent condition in the development of cancer (Snow, 1893; Evans, 1926; Blumberg, West and Ellis, 1954; Greene and Miller, 1958; LeShan, 1959, 1966; Renneker et al., 1963; Giovacchini and Muslin, 1965; Muslin, Gyarfas and Pieper, 1966; Priestman, Priestman and Bradshaw, 1985; Bahnson, 1969; Simonton and Simonton, 1975). A number of more recent studies claim to have demonstrated a link between stressful events and cancer (Schonfield, 1975; Stoll, 1979; Jacobs and Charles, 1980; Shekele et al., 1981; Rosch, 1984); and in the recurrence of cancer (Stoll, 1979; Alvarez, 1989), with the result that such a view is widely accepted and promoted (Cooper, Cooper and Eaker, 1988; Anonymous, 1987).

However, a number of studies have suggested that the attitude of the cancer patient is vitally important in determining the outcome of illness. Those patients whose cancer undergoes spontaneous remission have been found to be more positive in attitude. A clear correlation has been demonstrated between mental attitude and length of survival (Greer, Morris and Pettingdale, 1979). Similarly, those cancer patients who outlive predicted life expectancies have been found to refuse to give up in the face of stress (Achterberg, Simonton and Simonton,

1977). These findings are significant in the light of the discovery that expectation influences blood levels of the hormones cortisol and prolactin, which are important in activating the immune system (Breznitz, 1984). The subsequent realization that positive and negative expectations have opposite effects, respectively enhancing or depressing the immune response clearly has implications for treatment in general, and understanding of the placebo effect in particular.

Recognition of the importance of positive attitudes and expectations has led to the idea that positive emotions are not only life-enhancing but also immuno-enhancing experiences. This has largely come about as the result of the pioneering work of cancer specialist Carl Simonton and his wife Stephanie, a psychotherapist. Their approach, which combines insights derived from the fields of psychoneuroendocrinology, psychoneuroimmunology, meditative approaches and psychotherapy, rests on the theory that emotional and mental states play a significant role both in susceptibility and recovery from all disease, including cancer. They also note that both stress and the belief system of the cancer patient can be modified to good effect by way of relaxation and visualization. Accordingly, they argue (Simonton and Simonton, 1975) that the first step in getting well is to understand how psychological factors have contributed to illness and to find ways of influencing them in support of treatment.

They recognize that in helping to promote or enhance relaxation, imagery has an important role in decreasing tension and effecting positive physiological changes. These include improvement of immune function, and thus influence the course of malignancy. These techniques may be used to help patients confront their fears of hopelessness and helplessness, enabling them to gain a sense of control and change in attitude. They also provide a means of communication with their unconscious minds, where beliefs antithetical to health may be hidden, which may yield valuable insights into their condition.

Carl Simonton first taught his patients a simple form of relaxation focused on breathing. They were then instructed to repeat silently the word relax and to let go of tensions in various muscle complexes which are typically responsive to stress by focusing on them in turn. Once this was achieved they were encouraged to imagine a pleasant place and to hold this in mind. They were then asked to imagine their illness in any way it appeared to them, and the form of treatment they were receiving. Having done this, they were to imagine the cancer shrinking or otherwise responding in a positive way to treatment. The patients were also encouraged to imagine pain in the same way rather than trying to suppress it.

Of 159 patients with a diagnosis of medically incurable malignancy treated over a 4 year period, prior to 1978, none of whom were expected to live more than a year, 22.2% were reported (Simonton, Matthews-Simonton and Creighton, 1978) as having made a full recovery. The disease regressed in a further 17% of patients and stabilized in 27%. Further tumour growth was reported in 31% of the patients but average survival time increased by a factor of 1.5–2. Those who eventually succumbed to the malignancy were reported as having maintained higher than usual levels of activity, and achieved a significant improvement in their quality of life.

Abundant anecdotal evidence, including accounts by children (Gillespie, 1989), has since supported the Simontons' claim that relaxation and imagery have an important role to play in the treatment of cancer as adjuncts to orthodox medical treatment. Improved cancer outcome related to the uses of imagery has also been reported by Borysenko (1987). Support has also been forthcoming from a number of studies (Fiore, 1974; Meares, 1981) which confirm that visualization has numerous effects, including cancer regression. Guided imagery and visualization have been found to provide cancer patients with considerable relief from pain, nausea, vomiting, anticipatory emesis and anxiety (Donovan, 1980; Bradley and McCanne, 1981; Walker, reported in Harley, 1989); and to be effective in reducing the aversiveness of cancer chemotherapy (Lyles *et al.*, 1982).

Increasingly, contemporary practitioners of imaginative medicine are using imagery in diagnosis and treatment, and to relieve the pain and anxiety associated with medical conditions. Achterberg describes the pioneers of imaginative methods in modern medical practice as trying to bridge the gulf between the different worlds of magic and medical science, mind and body, and terms them 'shaman/scientists'. Arguably, however, such a term is highly misleading, because to a great extent modern practitioners ignore the spirit, which shamans traditionally consider the most important factor in disease, health and healing, as Achterberg acknowledges:

> The modern shaman/scientists, unlike their predecessors in the healing arts, typically do not claim to be operating within the transpersonal mode of imaginary healing. Rather, they are likely to envisage themselves as teachers or guides, with any healing or diagnostic benefit coming from the patient themselves. They can best be generalized as ascribing to the preverbal notion of healing with the imagination, regarding it as a natural, but often latent, human ability. Transpersonal healing may well be entertained by the shaman/scientist as viable in certain clinical applications, but it does not form the theoretical basis for the tools and techniques of the imagination that are currently being integrated into medical settings (Achterberg, 1985, p. 76).

Although there is still need for further carefully controlled studies, imaginative methods have been widely adopted in the USA and Europe, where they have been promoted enthusiastically by physicians such as Dossey (1982) and Siegel (1986, 1990). They have been promoted more cautiously by Sikora (reported in Harley, 1989) in Britain, where psychological approaches involving imagery have been introduced into a number of orthodox hospital cancer treatment programmes as doctors have come round to the view that these methods are compatible with traditional methods of treatment. Success has also been claimed for the effectiveness of imagery in the absence of orthodox medical treatments such as surgery, chemotherapy and radiography (Brohn, 1986), although there is no empirical evidence to support this.

Achterberg and Lawlis (1978) have researched and practised imagery techniques in a variety of health care settings for many years 'in the belief that the shamanic techniques that served the world so well in medicine since the beginning of recorded history should not be discarded but improved on' (Achterberg, 1985, pp. 101–2). They point out that the techniques have been validated on patients suffering from chronic pain, severe orthopaedic trauma, rheumatoid arthritis, cancer, diabetes, burn injury, alcoholism, stress disorders and childbirth. Moreover, a significant increase in NK activity, together with a decrease in antibodies to the herpes simplex virus suggestive of better control of the virus by the immune system, has been demonstrated in a controlled study of patients taught guided imagery techniques (Kiecolt-Glaser et al., 1985).

Evidence for immunoenhancement has also been demonstrated in response to essentially image-based stimuli such as humour (Cousins, 1981a), humorous (Dillon, Minchoff and Baker, 1985) and compassionate films (McClelland and Kirschnit, 1984). In the latter study, subjects exposed to a film about Mother Theresa's work caring for the sick and poor showed increased IGA levels regardless of whether they outwardly approved of her work or not. These results suggest that information and suggestions can be acquired by subjects unconsciously and may enhance immune function whether or not the subjects are aware of an effect or emotional reaction. Positive and immune enhancing imagery techniques have also shown specific immunological consequences. Hypnotized subjects, who were encouraged to imagine their white blood cells as sharks attacking the germs in their body, showed an actual increase in the number of lymphocytes (Hall, Longo and Dixon, 1981). Taken together these studies suggest the possibility of increasing the ability to enhance and control the immune system through conscious or unconscious suggestion, or by exposure to positively enhancing stimuli. Interventions with imagery may therefore prevent, or at least delay, the progress of AIDS in seropositive males (Coates and Greenblatt, 1986). Anecdotal support for the role of imaginative interventions in the treatment of AIDS is also provided by Asistent and Duffy (1991). However, one of the most significant studies in this area (Smith et al., 1985) has demonstrated voluntary regulation of a specific immune function through imagery by a subject. Norris (1989) observes that such findings are consistent with the earlier research findings on biofeedback of Pelletier and Peper (1977) which provided the first unequivocal evidence that adept meditators could voluntarily control pain, bleeding and infection from self-induced puncture wounds.

Taken together, the findings in this rapidly growing and exciting field of psychoneuroimmunology, have important implications for imaginative medicine. As Achterberg (1985) points out, in order for the imagination to move from its current adjunctive role in medicine and be awarded the stature achieved in the shamanic system of healing, the role of the imagination in total health must be supported by a body of solid, convincing research. 'This is the area in which the research on the role of the imagination in health has been most clearly delineated using scientific method' (Achterberg, 1985, p. 161).

Modern developments in imaginative medicine: 'psychophysics'

4

> Imagination is more important than education.
> *Albert Einstein*

Pelletier and Herzing (1989, p. 379) conclude their review of recent develop-ments in psychoneuroimmunology with the observation that 'data from the emerging field of psychoneuroimmunology and related disciplines increasingly indicate a mind–body continuum and discredit the anachronistic split of Cartesian dualism'. Moreover, the growing recognition within these fields of the influence of various psychosocial factors on immunity (Dohrenwend, 1974; Grossarth-Maticek, Bastians and Kanazin, 1985; Baltrusch and Waltz, 1986), such as social support (Broadhead *et al.*, 1983; Wills, 1985; Roos and Cohen, 1987; Ganster and Victor, 1988); and social interactions (Pilisik and Parks, 1986; Roos and Cohen, 1987; Sarason, Sarason and Pierce, 1988; Grassi and Lodi, 1989; Speigel *et al.*, 1989); including human-animal relationships (Mugford and McComisky, 1975; Holden, 1981; Arehart-Treichel, 1982; McCulloch, 1982; Friedmann *et al.*, 1982, 1983; Arkow, 1984; Grossberg and Alf, 1984; Serpell, 1990, 1991) highlights the fact that organisms can no longer be considered in isolation from each other, different species, or their environ-ment. This awareness has led to the emergence of a new discipline which acknowledges the unitary ontological nature of reality. It focuses attention not only on interactions between the neurological, psychological and immunologi-cal aspects of being but also between the biological and social, viewing them as 'neither separable, nor antithetical, nor alternatives, but complementary' (Rose, Kamin and Lewontin, 1984, pp. 273–4). This so-called 'new biology' is consis-tent with a not-so-new understanding of reality; a radically different model which totally undermines the Cartesian/Newtonian notion of a clockwork universe, and has led to its abandonment during the twentieth century. The key figure in this conceptual revolution was Albert Einstein.

THE UNCERTAIN UNIVERSE OF ALBERT EINSTEIN

Einstein (1879–1955) dealt a major blow to the notion of a clockwork universe with the publication in 1905 of his *Theory of Special Relativity*. This effectively shifted understanding of the universe from a model that was mechanistic and deterministic to one that is relativistic and uncertain. It did so by presenting radically different concepts of space and time to those which are the basis of traditional or classical Newtonian physics. In relativity theory space is not three-dimensional and time is not a separate entity. One cannot therefore consider time without space. Both are intimately connected, forming a four-dimensional continuum of space–time, which can be mapped or represented diagrammatically as a network of interrelated events which have no definite direction of time attached to them. Hence there is no before or after in the processes they picture and thus no linear relationship of cause or effect, unless direction is imposed on the 'map' by reading it in a certain way, say from bottom to top. All events are interconnected but the connections between them are not causal in the Newtonian sense, and so, depending on how a person accesses the map or picture, ordering of events will be different. There is thus no universal flow of time as in the Newtonian model and this has startling implications.

Different observers will order events differently, depending on their point of view. Therefore, two events seen as occurring simultaneously by one observer may occur in different temporal sequence for other observers. Accordingly the concept of a universal and absolute standard of public time divided into past, present and future is an illusion. The idea of subjective time, with its focus on 'now', has no objective meaning because the past and future exist and are equally real in the present; events are simply there in space-time, and do not happen. It would seem, therefore, that what moves or flows, is not time, but the human mind.

In 1915, Einstein extended the special theory of relativity to include gravity. The resulting general theory of relativity described the large-scale structure of the universe. The picture was totally different than that conceived by Newton, which was based on the notion of solid material bodies moving in empty space.

In Einstein's formulation any distinction between mass and energy is abandoned. Mass and energy are simply different manifestations of each other, mass being a bound form of energy. His famous equation $E=mc^2$ (where E is energy, m is mass and c *is* the speed of light) is the mathematical statement of the equivalence of mass and energy; that mass has energy and energy has mass, and that the energy that an object has owing to its motion will add to its mass. Therefore mass is no longer associated with a material substance and is not seen as consisting of any basic 'stuff', but as bundles or quanta of energy. As energy is associated with activity, and with processes, this implies that the nature of matter is intrinsically dynamic. Thus, matter can no longer be pictured as composed of units, such as tiny billiard balls or grains of sand, as in the

Newtonian view. It has to be understood as dynamic patterns of activity which have a spatial and a temporal aspect; the former making them appear as objects with a certain mass, and the latter making them appear as processes involving the equivalent energy. In Einstein's view therefore, the being of matter and its activity are different aspects of the same space–time reality and cannot be separated.

The equivalence of mass and energy has since been verified innumerable times, forcing a fundamental modification of existing notions. However, the Newtonian concept is so ingrained in Western thought that these changes have not been easily accommodated. In 1909, when Rutherford split the atom, it became clear that atoms were not the solid objects conceived by Newton. They are vast regions of empty space in which extremely small particles (electrons) move around a nucleus, bound to it by electric forces. The distinction between matter and empty space finally had to be abandoned when it became evident that particles can come into being spontaneously out of the void and vanish again into it.

Further astonishing discoveries resulted from investigations into the subatomic realm in the early twentieth century. In the 1920s it was found that subatomic particles make discontinuous jumps or quantum leaps from one orbit to another, without leaving any trace of their path. What became known as quantum theory, holds that a particle, such as an electron, does not have a meaningful trajectory but abrupt and unpredictable motion. Thus, at the subatomic level, matter does not exist with certainty at definite places, nor do atomic events occur with certainty at definite times and in definite ways. Rather, matter shows 'tendencies to exist' and subatomic events show 'tendencies to occur', which can be expressed mathematically as probabilities in the form of waves. Subsequently the mathematical formulation of quantum theory (quantum mechanics) imposed order on this apparent chaos or entropy by giving the probabilities of when and where a particle might be. Atomic events can therefore never be predicted with certainty, only the likelihood of their happening.

Such a view completely overturns common sense. Einstein preferred the common sense view that electrons really exist in a definite place and with a definite trajectory, maintaining that any ambiguity or uncertainty encountered in the observation of atoms is the result of imprecision in the measuring instruments used. However the 'common sense' view was subsequently shown to be false.

Logically it does not seem possible that something can at one and the same time be both a particle and a wave. The Danish physicist and Nobel laureate Niels Bohr (1885–1962) resolved this curious paradox by suggesting that the particle and wave pictures are two complementary and mutually exclusive descriptions of the same reality, both of which are necessary. In so doing, he highlighted the inadequacy of concepts such as waves and particles in describing atomic phenomena. Subsequently it was recognized that an electron is neither a particle nor a wave, but can show aspects of either depending on how it is observed.

THE UNCERTAINTY PRINCIPLE

The German physicist Werner Heisenberg (1901–1976) established that there are limits beyond which the processes of nature cannot be measured accurately as they are taking place. There are limits beyond which there can be no certainty, and that are not imposed by the inexactness of measuring devices or the extremely small size of the entities being measured, but by nature itself.

> The uncertainty principle reveals that as we penetrate deeper and deeper into the subatomic realm, we reach a certain point at which one part or another of our picture of nature becomes blurred, and there is no way to reclarify that part without blurring another part of the picture! It is as though we are adjusting a moving picture that is slightly out of focus. As we make the final adjustments we are astonished to discover that when the right side of the picture clears, the left side of the picture becomes completely unfocused and nothing in it is recognizable. When we try to focus the left side of the picture, the right side starts to blur and soon the situation is reversed.

> If we try to strike a balance between these two extremes, both sides of the picture return to a recognizable condition, but in no way can we remove the original fuzziness from them. The right side of the picture, in the original formulation of the uncertainty principle, corresponds to the position in space of a moving article. The left side of the picture corresponds to its momentum. According to the uncertainty principle, we cannot measure accurately at the same time, both the position and the momentum of a moving particle. The more precisely we determine one of these properties the less we know about the other. If we precisely determine the position of the particle, then, strange as it sounds, there is nothing that we can know about its momentum. If we precisely determine the momentum of the particle, there is no way to determine its position (Zukav, 1980, p. 133).

The primary significance of the uncertainty principle is that all attempts to observe the electron alter it, so at the subatomic level it is not possible to observe something without changing it. Therefore, reality does not exist independently of the observer who measures it. Indeed the uncertainty principle suggests that reality is actually shaped by the observer.

> My conscious decision about how to observe say an electron will determine the electron's properties to some extent. If I ask it a particle question it will give me a particle answer; if I ask it a wave question it will give me a wave answer. The electron does not have objective properties independent of mind (Capra, 1982a, p. 7).

By dispensing with the notion of a fixed, observable reality, the uncertainty principle signified the end of a completely predictable universe. As Hawking (1988, p. 55) observes, 'One certainly cannot predict future events exactly if one cannot even measure the present state of the universe precisely!'. It follows therefore that the Newtonian ideal of a measurable objectivity in science is totally unfounded. Once again, as 'the concrete matter of daily experience dissolves into a maelstrom of fleeting ghostly images' (Pagels, 1983, p. 102) the implications seem bizarre, but as Niels Bohr observed, 'those who aren't shocked by quantum theory have not understood it'.

Einstein was disturbed by many of the discoveries of quantum physics, particularly those of Heisenberg, and so in 1935 with Boris Podolsky and Nathan Rosen, he devised an argument which he believed to be the *reductio ad absurdem* of quantum theory. This Einstein–Podolsky–Rosen theorem essentially proposed that if quantum theory is correct, then a change in the spin of a two particle system should affect its twin simultaneously, even if the two were widely separated, This implies some form of telepathic communication or psychokinesis – physical action at a distance. This represented an unthinkable proposition for most physicists of the time who regarded telepathy and psychokinesis as occultist nonsense, including Einstein who regarded the idea as 'ghostly and absurd'.

However, in 1964, J.S. Bell formulated a mathematical proof, subsequently known as Bell's theorem, which suggested that Einstein's improbable proposition of action at a distance could occur. This was confirmed experimentally in 1972 and the findings have been replicated on numerous occasions since. In 1983, a French team of scientists led by Alain Aspect added a crucial refinement to previous experiments that established beyond doubt that as far as action at a distance is concerned, quantum theory was right and Einstein wrong.

Aspect's experiment has dramatic implications for physics. One possible conclusion to be drawn from it is that some kind of information can travel faster than the speed of light. This means that existing concepts of space and time require modification; or it may mean that everything in the universe is interrelated and interconnected.

> No matter how formulated, it projects the 'irrational' aspects of subatomic phenomena squarely into the macroscopic domain. It says that not only do events in the realm of the small behave in ways which are utterly different from our common sense view of the world but also that events in the world at large, the world of freeways and sports cars, behave in ways which are utterly different from our common sense view of them (Zukav, 1980, p. 306).

Bell's theorem resonates with the theories of Carl Jung, who argued for the interconnectedness of all things in an essay written in collaboration with the physicist Wolfgang Pauli (Jung, 1972b). Here Jung used the term synchronicity to describe the simultaneous occurrence of two meaningfully but not causally related events, or the timely coincidence of two or more unrelated events with the same or similar meaning. Heutzer (1984) suggests that this concept is a modern derivation of the mystical and magical belief in the fundamental unity of all things. He notes that since antiquity, influences, sympathies and correspondences have been invoked as explanations for events that seem unaffected by causal laws. This doctrine of the 'sympathy of all things' can be traced back to Hippocrates, and is a recurrent theme in Western philosophy until the eighteenth century, when following the Newtonian revolution 'causality was enthroned as the absolute ruler of matter and mind' (Heutzer, 1984, pp. 89–90). It was this reign that quantum theory brought to an abrupt end.

> If all actions are in the form of discrete quanta, the interactions between different entities (e.g. electrons) constitute a single structure of indivisible links, so that the entire universe has to be thought of as an unbroken whole. In this whole, each element that we can extract in thought shows basic properties (wave or particle etc.) that depend on its overall environment in a way that is much more reminiscent of how the organs constituting living things are related, than it is of how parts of a machine interact. Further the non-local, non-causal nature of the relationships of elements distant from each other violates the requirements of separateness and independence of fundamental constituents that is basic to any mechanistic approach (Bohm, 1980, pp. 175–6).

Modern physics therefore suggests that at a deep and fundamental level the apparently separate parts of the universe are connected in an intimate and immediate way. Indeed the organic, holistic, ecological world view which has emerged in the twentieth century restates, albeit in the language of mathematics, occult and mystical descriptions of reality in evidence since antiquity, and still emphasized within Eastern cultures.

CONVERGENCE BETWEEN PHYSICS AND MYSTICISM

The striking parallels between the discoveries of modern physicists and Eastern mystics have been identified by numerous commentators, including LeShan (1969, 1974). A thorough discussion of the correspondences between the theories of subatomic and atomic physics and Taoist thought, in particular, has been provided by Capra (1976) and Zukav (1980). Certainly, as Capra points out, Bohr and Heisenberg were well aware of this correspondence, as are leading modern physicists such as David Bohm. Initially, however, many physicists reared in the Newtonian tradition were shocked at any comparison between physics and mysticism. Increasingly, physicists are becoming aware that mysticism provides a consistent and relevant philosophical background to the theories of contemporary science.

The undivided wholeness they imply, in which all parts of the universe, including the observer and all instruments, merge and unite in one interdependent totality demands a fundamentally different conceptualization of the way in which the universe is arranged or ordered. The mechanistic order may be described as a system in which each of its elements lies only in its own regions of space and time and outside the regions appertaining to other things. It is in this sense that events are conceived as separate and independent, and are understandable in terms of the regular arrangements of objects, as in rows, or events in sequence.

Bohm (1980) has proposed a concept of order appropriate to the undivided wholeness implied by quantum theory. He suggests that the universe is like a giant hologram in which information about the whole is contained implicitly in each of its parts so that if broken into pieces each will reconstruct the whole. However, a hologram is essentially a static record of this implicate order, which is conveyed in a complex movement of electromagnetic fields in the form of light waves. Bohm therefore uses the term holomovement to describe the unbroken and undivided totality or life energy from which particular aspects, such as light and sound or electrons, may be abstracted, but from which they cannot be separated. In Bohm's theory therefore, the fundamental reality is movement, and the world of manifest reality is a secondary derivation from this primary order of the universe. The 'hard' reality and facts so esteemed within traditional scientific theory and method are therefore an abstraction from the 'blur' of basic reality, a notion long held by mystics and sages and reflected in the teachings of Gibran's prophet:

> Life, and all that lives, is conceived in the mist and not in the crystal. And
> who knows but a crystal is a mist in decay (Gibran, 1978, pp. 108–9).

Like the mystics of antiquity, Bohm, in describing a holographic universe, is depicting a world in which what appears to be stable, tangible and 'out there' is not really there at all, and is thus an illusion, a magic show. In the terms of Indian philosophy it is maya. Such a view has also been advanced by the neuroscientist Karl Pribram (1978). He suggests that reality is not what is perceived by the eyes, but that the brain acts as a lens, mathematically transforming the blur of primary reality into 'hard' reality. Without these mathematics, we would possibly only know a world organized in the frequency domain; a world without space or time, such as that described by poets and mystics throughout history, where 'what is essential is invisible to the eye' (St. Exupéry, 1974).

Nevertheless, the problem for the physicist and neuroscientist is to account for 'normal' perception of mundane 'explicate' reality; that which Indian sages term avidja (a not-seeing). Castaneda's tutor, Don Juan, claims that 'we train our eyes to look as we think about the things we look at; so in essence the world that your reason wants to sustain is the world created by a description and its dogmatic and inviolable rules which the reason learns to accept and defend'.

He argues that true 'seeing' demands suspension of thought, reason and logic. Similarly Bohm suggests that humans learn to see the world in certain ways, and because they are habituated to the explicate order which is emphasized in thought and language, both of which are predominantly linear and sequential, they do not ordinarily notice the primary order. Indeed Western culture as a whole is habituated to the rational, the logical, the linear and sequential, and to a description of a manifest, explicate reality. As a result the ability to 'think straight' is highly valued and there is a tendency to feel that primary experience is of that order. Another possible reason for this oversight, according to Bohm, is that the contents of memory, in the manner of a holograph, focus attention on what is static and fragmented. Thus, the more subtle and transitory features of the unbroken flow 'tend to pale into such seeming insignificance that one is at best only dimly conscious of them' (Bohn, 1980, p. 208).

Mystical traditions emphasize that true seeing, or direct perception of reality, can be achieved by the development of insight, literally a looking inwards. This is consistent with the holographic notion that the world is implicitly enfolded within each of its parts. Accordingly, the truth of the universe, ultimate truth, resides within the person:

> The things we see...are the things which are already in us. There is no reality beyond what we have inside us (Hermann Hesse, *Demian*).

The literature of mysticism, which claims that by looking inwards one encounters nothingness (variously referred to as pure or cosmic consciousness, Brahman, Atman or the universal Tao) bears an uncanny resemblance to the descriptions of reality offered by quantum theory. The contents of this experience are often said to be 'ineffable', or incapable of being fully expressed in words, but Huxley (1977) indicates that there are similarities in attempts to do so. Undifferentiated, uncoloured light is commonly referred to; as is the experience of light in differentiated forms, when it is embodied in shapes, landscapes and personages. Huxley claims that this visionary world (the world seen with what he terms the 'inner eye', and which bears a striking resemblance to the archetypal world of the collective unconscious described by Jung) is accessed in various ways. These include hypnosis, various forms of meditation, total isolation and sensory deprivation, breathing exercises, fasting, drugs and other substances which have been used in mystical, magical and shamanic practices from the earliest times, and more recently by scientists such as William James, John Lilly and Stanislav Grof in their explorations of consciousness. These drugs, it would seem, prevent the individual from 'thinking straight' and bypass what Huxley has termed the 'reducing valve' of ordinary consciousness, enabling direct perception of reality; the undifferentiated frequency domain postulated by Bohm and Pribram. This is a view supported by Grof (1979) who argues that psychedelic drugs, facilitate access to the holographic universe they have described.

In the light of these speculations, concern with mystical experience and altered states of consciousness can no longer be dismissed as trivial. These phenomena have to be admitted within any scientific framework purporting to be a complete understanding of reality. Certainly the emergent paradigm afforded by modern physics admits consciousness in a previously unconceived way. It implies, in contradistinction to common sense views of reality, that it may not be the brain that produces consciousness or mind, but rather consciousness that creates the appearance of the brain, matter, space, time and everything that is taken as constituting the physical universe. Given such a possibility, consciousness must be considered and explored in any attempt at understanding the universe and man's place in it. Indeed, as Polanyi (1958) has indicated, any science attempting a strictly detached, objective knowledge and to abolish all personal knowledge would be aiming, unwittingly, at the destruction of all knowledge. The ideal of science would thus turn out to be fundamentally misleading and possibly the source of devastating fallacies.

It is ironic, therefore, that at the very time scientists were awakening to the possibility that the universe is more akin to mind than machine, psychology, in its insistence on so-called objective fact, was rejecting all subjective phenomena as unscientific and denying the very existence of consciousness. The absurdity of the situation was highlighted by Koestler (1976, p. 32):

> Materialism is 'vieux jeux', a century out of date. Only you psychologists still believe in it. It is a very funny situation. We know that the behaviour of an electron is not completely determined by the laws of physics. You believe that the behaviour of a human being is completely determined by the laws of physics. Electrons are unpredictable, people are predictable. And you call this psychology.

Indeed, as Hearnshaw indicates, despite the fact that the physics which had served as a model for late nineteenth century psychology has been almost totally transformed, psychologists continued slavishly to adhere to it up until at least the middle of the twentieth century. Yet the implications of the new physics for psychology are considerable:

> The human mind is, of course, adapted primarily to dealing with a middle-scale world, and for practical purposes the psychologist must consider its adjustment to this world. But the middle-scale world has now almost vanished between the infinitely small and the infinitely large. Within it no stable basis for theory remains, and beyond it common sense generalizations no longer apply (Hearnshaw, 1989, pp. 227–8).

Psychological theory and methodology need rethinking accordingly, but as Hearnshaw indicates, 'Psychologists, particularly the new breed of twentieth century academic psychologists, were remarkably slow to respond to these challenges. Many of them were more interested in experimentation on rats and other animals, where old-fashioned methodology could be applied, than in considering the difficult problems of human psychology' (Hearnshaw, 1989, p. 228).

CONSCIOUSNESS AND TRANSFORMATION

One of the most difficult problems for psychology, working within the frame-work of a materialistic, mechanistic paradigm, is in generating consciousness from an impersonal universe. Psychology had unsatisfactorily resolved this problem during the first half of the twentieth century by ignoring, and even denying, the existence of consciousness. Cosgrove (1982) argues the case for materialism in psychology by insisting that humanistic psychology, in attempt-ing to justify the existence of consciousness when the material world cannot produce it, is building its view of human nature on a presuppositional basis that will not support such a lofty view of man. He insists that 'this is not just a biological problem that will some day be solved. Trying to draw more from nature than it has to give demands a suspension of logic that scientists make in no other part of their work' (p. 73). In the light of the new physics this assertion is patently untrue. Moreover it fails to take into account the contributions of the distinguished chemist, Ilya Prigogine.

In 1977, Prigogine was awarded the Nobel prize for his transformation theory which established the connectedness of living and non-living forms, and thus bridged the critical gap between living systems and the apparently lifeless universe in which they arise. Prigogine recognizes his theory as being consistent with the visions of poets, mystics and Eastern philosophers of an open, creative universe.

Prigogine's theory concerns dissipative structures, this includes all living things and some non-living things, such as certain chemical reactions the form of which is maintained by a continuing dissipation of energy. As such they constitute a flowing wholeness which is highly complex and always in process. The greater their complexity, the more energy such structures require to main-tain coherence, which produces the paradoxical situation whereby the greater their coherence the greater their instability. However, Prigogine suggests that this instability is the key to transformation because the dissipation of energy creates the potential for sudden re-ordering and reorganization.

> The continuous movement of energy through the system results in fluctu-ations; if they are minor the system damps them and they do not alter its structural integrity. But if the fluctuations reach a critical size they 'perturb' the system. They increase the number of novel interactions within it. They shake it up. The elements of the old pattern come into contact with each other in new ways and make new connections. The parts reorganize into a new whole. The system escapes to a higher order.

> The more complex or coherent a structure, the greater the next level of complexity. Each new level is even more integrated and connected than the one before, requiring a greater flow of energy for maintenance, and is therefore still less stable. To put it another way, flexibility begets flexibil-ity. As Prigogine said, at higher levels of complexity, 'the nature of the

laws of nature changes'. It has the potential to create new forms by allowing a shake-up of old forms (Ferguson, 1983, p. 178).

Paradoxically, it is instability, or the capacity for being 'shaken up' which is the key to growth. Perturbation is therefore bound up in shifts towards physiological complexity. Structures insulated from it and protected from change, stagnate and never evolve toward a more complex form.

TRANSFORMATION AND HEALTH

Viewed within the framework of transformation theory, disease is clearly a perturbation. Accordingly, it is a means whereby the system can, in Prigogine's terms, 'escape' to a higher level of organization or integration, and thus achieve greater wholeness or health. Dossey (1982) observes that the tenets of transformation theory are already invoked in many health-care methodologies including orthodox medical practice. Immunization, for example, involves inducing a mini-disease just sufficient to stimulate the body to produce protective antibodies, thereby 'producing an evolution toward biological complexity through intentionally perturbing the immune system' (p. 89). He suggests that if perturbation of the body's integration never occurred it would be totally defenceless, because necessary mechanisms would not evolve. This is the case with children born with immune deficiency, who because they are unable to respond to perturbations from outside cannot escape to a higher degree of immune complexity and usually succumb to overwhelming infections early in life.

Clearly, therefore, the processes of perturbation or dis-ease and health form a complementary whole. However, as Dossey indicates, orthodox medicine frequently moves against perturbation rather than with it, 'battering the perceived threats with a constantly changing array of injections, pills and surgery', and trying 'to avoid encounters with external challenges to our health; failing that, we struggle to resist them using any means at hand' (Dossey, 1982, p. 91).

Indeed the institution of medicine itself reflects this resistance to external challenges by adhering steadfastly to an outmoded model of how the world behaves and almost totally ignoring the insights of modern physics. The result is that medicine finds itself 'with a set of guiding beliefs that are as antiquated as are body humors, leeching and bleeding' (Dossey, 1982, p. xii). Like psychology, medicine has built its concepts of the body, health, illness, birth and death on the model of Newtonian physics, and resisted any redefinition of these notions. It is still governed by mechanistic thinking, the body being viewed essentially as a machine in good or bad repair, disease or disability as a thing or entity to be treated by elimination of symptoms, primarily with drugs and surgery after diagnosis, which relies on quantitative information. Psychological factors, where acknowledged at all, are regarded as of secondary importance, with psychosomatic illness treated by a separate specialism, psychiatry. All treatment, however, is viewed as a matter for professionals who are emotionally neutral authority figures, responsible for patients who are passive and dependent.

The radical reformulation of reality provided by modern physics is profoundly unsettling to those attached to the old scientific paradigm, demanding as it does a fundamental re-examination of the principles and practices of medicine. However such crises are a precondition for the emergence of a new perspective, because it is only as a result of these changes that scientific understanding develops. Without some shaking of their foundations, as indicated in transformation theory, systems of knowledge cannot evolve and progress. Hence the history of science is characterized by such shifts. The implications for medicine of continuing to resist the challenge they offer are therefore considerable, for as Dossey (1989, p. 400) observes, 'Flawed images of the body lead to flawed therapies for the body'.

The fundamental problem facing contemporary medicine is to reconcile ordinary 'common sense' descriptions of bodies, health and disease with the idea of quantum wholeness. While this does not mean that these notions cannot be abstracted as apparently discrete features of reality, and spoken of as aspects of the world (in just the way that physicists speak of the wave and particle features of electrons), it does mean that cognisance has to be taken of the underlying unbroken wholeness that envelopes all manifestations of the entire universe.

When translated into practice these new conceptions of reality require bodies, health and disease to be viewed as dynamic processes instead of discrete entities. They need to be understood in terms of patterns and relationships within the organism and its environment, rather than in terms of symptoms, or the lack of them. Accordingly, mind has to be regarded as a primary factor in health and illness and therefore so-called 'psychosomatic illness' becomes a matter for all health care professionals, who are therapeutic partners in the healing process rather than external to it. Essentially, therefore, the new description of reality demands, as did Hippocrates, that physicians understand 'the whole of things'.

Indeed the insights provided by transformation theory are far from new. In ancient Greece, theatre was recognized and valued as therapy because of its power to 'shake up' or perturb. The Greeks believed that the evocation of unsettling emotions such as fear and pity, by tragedy caused a profound change to take place; an emotional purging or purification, which Aristotle termed catharsis.

> The assumption is that the emotional stresses within us, often subconscious, and the moral contradictions too, likely to be equally deeply buried, need to be relieved and resolved. By losing our everyday awareness of ourselves and by identifying with the actors – themselves divested of self in the drama's heightened world – we expose ourselves to the full force of their sufferings and sins as we may never be able to admit to our own, and thus effect relief... Aristotle thought that to witness tragedy in a theatre is one of the ways in which human beings can be purged of stress

and inner conflict. Our own pity and fear draw us towards a point of balance, he believed, and from this comes a sense of health, and therefore pleasure.

The Greeks believed that life was to be enjoyed, but they also knew its pains and terrors, and their own vulnerability to its dark and irrational forces. Tragedy was a means to contain and express the paradox, but it was also an end in itself, the creation of something for the living even out of death (Harwood, 1984, pp. 53–4).

The Greeks also understood that laughter could possess and purge an audience, and comedy was therefore widely used as therapy several thousand years before its healing effects were pointed to by Cousins (1981a), Holden (1992) and Dillon, Minchoff and Baker (1985). Humour was also of central importance in the teachings of the Buddha, who in Indian tradition is depicted as the enlightened one, who, being able to see the folly of man's habitual attachment to intellect and ego and the resulting deception as to the true nature of reality, laughs at this huge cosmic joke. The importance of humour is emphasized by other Indian masters who insist, like Rajneesh (1979), that 'humour will join your split parts, glue your fragments into one whole'; that seriousness is a blocked stage of mind, a state of 'unflow' or stagnancy; and that serious people are therefore ill people. There is also considerable levity, hilarity and humour in the shamanic tradition as recounted by Carlos Castaneda.

Similarly, an understanding of trauma as a means of creating new order by perturbation is paralleled in numerous ways within traditional systems of knowledge. Teachings of the Buddha emphasize the possibility of transformation through acceptance of change and direct confrontation with the anxieties it generates. Certain practices, such as a Zen master striking his pupil, enable him to 'see' the truth of a paradoxical koan. In these traditional systems, transformation is achieved primarily as a result of powerful sensations evoked by imagery during meditation and visionary experience. In effecting a 'shake-up' of existing assumptions and views of the world, imagery yields new and significant insights, suggests different possibilities and enables problems to be transformed into solutions. While this has been recognized in Eastern traditions, it has only recently been understood in the West, as a result of psychological research into human cognition and problem solving.

Perturbation or 'shake-up' of existing assumptions and perceptions may similarly account for the transformative effects claimed for psychotherapy:

> An individual reliving a traumatic incident in a state of highly-focused inward attention perturbs the pattern of that specific old memory. This triggers a reorganization – a new dissipative structure. The old pattern is broken (Ferguson, 1983, p. 183).

Furthermore, it has been advanced as a possible explanation of mental illness by the psychiatrist R.D. Laing (1959), who suggested that mental 'dis-order' facilitates the reintegration of the personal self, and by Jourard (1971). Indeed regarding 'self' as a dissipative structure helps to account for many of the effects Jung claimed for psychotherapy. Insofar as Jung saw order and reintegration arising spontaneously out of disorder and chaos through a process of self-organization, his views are similar to those of Prigogine. Indeed in describing the psyche Jung used concepts which parallel those of modern physics.

PARALLELS BETWEEN JUNGIAN PSYCHOLOGY AND MODERN PHYSICS

In Jung's psychology everything is dynamic, subject to change; only the most important perspectives, only the basic principles are unalterable. The rest, like the psyche itself, is subject to the Heraclitan principle that everything flows (Jacobi, 1962, p. xi).

Jung viewed all processes as energetic and, just as in modern physics there can be no direct perception of the subatomic realm, only inference of the existence of waves and particles from their effects, so the unconscious can only be known indirectly through images and symbols encountered in dreams, fantasies and visions. Similarly the psyche is not confined to space and time. Jung insisted that only ignorance denies this fact, and that when the psyche is not under obligation to live in time and space, as in dreams and fantasy, it is not subject to these laws. This space–time awareness is apparent in his work on the concept of synchronicity, and his collaboration in this venture with the physicist Wolfgang Pauli reflects his belief that physics and psychology would have to draw together, because from different directions they map the same reality or transcendent territory. He believed that eventually they would arrive at agreement between psychological and physical concepts and achieve thereby a mind–body, spirit–matter synthesis. Therefore, if, as Watts (1961, p. 19) observed, there is no Einstein of the mind, Jung comes very close to being it.

IMAGINATIVE SCIENCE

Both Jung and Einstein focused attention on the importance of mental imagery, albeit in quite different ways, leading Inglis (1987, p. 241) to conclude:

By a weird twist of fate, it is beginning to look as if the quantum physicists are going to be regenerators of mind, overturning matter as their deity. And in the process, they have been going some way towards rehabilitating trance.

Indeed, Einstein's friend and biographer Antonia Vallentin recalled seeing him enter into a state 'not unlike the ecstasy of a saint'. Einstein admitted that his paper on the electrodynamics of bodies in movement, which foreshadowed his theory of relativity, originated in *gedanken* or 'thought' experiments. During them he realized that the stationary spatial oscillation he 'saw' when imagining himself travelling alongside a beam of light corresponded neither to anything that could be perceptually experienced as light, nor to anything described in existing mathematical equations. Hence the resulting paper contained no source references or citations from authorities (Inglis, 1990).

Einstein told various friends that the gift of fantasy meant more to him than any talent for absorbing information, and that his formulae were not derived from research or calculation but from 'psychical entities' reaching him as 'more or less clear images', some visual, and others 'of a muscular type'. He claimed that his ability lay chiefly in 'visualizing...effects, consequences and possibilities' (Holton, 1972, p. 110) rather than mathematics. Inglis observes that at the time Einstein was presenting his theories, these accounts would have been rejected as malicious misrepresentation, so strong was the assumption that scientists achieved their results through rational, logical processes. However, Einstein later confirmed these details quite explicitly in a letter to his biographer Jacques Hadamard, who, in his study of mathematicians (Hadamard, 1945) found that they too often relied on imagery in much the same way.

Subsequently, it has become clear that quantum physicists such as Eddington, Planck, Schroedinger, Heisenberg and others relied heavily on both imagination and intuition in the formulation of their theories. All appear to have regarded creative imagination as essential to scientific endeavour. Max Planck claimed that the scientist must possess 'a vivid, intuitive imagination', and Richard Feynman disclosed in a televised interview (1993), 'The game I play is this one: imagination in accordance with the laws of physics', laws, which to a great extent, have been established by way of the imagination.

Uncovering the mysteries of the universe by way of imagination has traditionally been the preserve of the mystic, and mastery over universal forces that of the magician, sorcerer or shaman. Wheatley (1973) has suggested that their art was the application of scientific laws which, for the most part, are still unknown to modern scientists. LeShan (1974) has also noted the similarity in world view between modern physicists and mystics. More recently this has been highlighted by Wilber (1984), who comments that from their writings (extracts from which he presents) Einstein, Eddington, Planck, Shrödinger and Heisenberg could all be taken for mystics. Moreover, this characteristic is not confined to quantum physicists.

Hadamard indicates that it was Faraday's ability to see in his inner eye which guided him to the invention of the dynamo and electric motor. His successor, James Clerk Maxwell, also reported having developed the habit of 'making a mental picture of every problem' (Beveridge, 1957, p. 56), and arriving at his formal equations only at the end of a series of elaborately visualized models. Tesla, the electrical engineer who developed the transformer, generator and dynamo, also used imagery to experiment with his inventions, in his mind rather than the laboratory. In this way he 'saw' the alternating current, the self-starting induction motor and the polyphase electrical system on which it depends, in the form of vivid imagery of a rotating magnetic field (Hunt and Draper, 1964). Spatial imagery also features strongly in geometrical conceptions of the complex electric and magnetic fields underlying the invention of the cyclotron, for which E.O. Lawrence was awarded the Nobel prize, and the alternating gradient synchrotron developed by Nicholas Christofilos (Shepard, 1977). Imagery has therefore played quite a significant role in the development of electromagnetic field theory in physics. It has also featured significantly in the development of the theory of molecular structures and its applications.

The German chemist, Fredrich Kekulé, claimed that his insights into the nature of the chemical bond, which form the basis of molecular theory, arose from spontaneous kinetic visual images. His cultivation of visionary practice culminated in his celebrated dream in which the image of a snake-like writhing molecule chain suddenly twisting into a closed loop, as if seizing its own tail, prompted him to solve the problem of the structure of benzine, which is fundamental to modern organic chemistry. McClintock solved the problems of the cycling of *Neurospora*, which had baffled distinguished geneticists for years, in the same way. Shepard observes that not only did imagery lead to the cracking of the genetic code by Watson in 1968, but is also crucial to the everyday work of chemists.

Hadamard (1945) suggested that the construction of verbal or symbolic outputs may also be guided by non-verbal images of schemata that capture what he termed 'the physiognomy of the problem'. There are clear indications that this is frequently the case in various forms of literary endeavour and creativity. Indeed it is well established that imagery is important to much creative output (Inglis, 1987). Charles Dickens (quoted in McKellar, 1968) insisted, 'I don't invent it, really do not, but 'see' it and write it down'. Similarly, Robert Louis Stevenson, Lewis Carroll and Wordsworth all acknowledged the importance of their capacity for imagery. Coleridge's claim that when writing his poem Kubla Khan 'all of the images rose up before him as things', bears a striking resemblance to Faraday's description of electric and magnetic fields in terms of images which 'rose up before him like things' (Ghiselin, 1952, p. 85). The poems of William Blake originated in much the same way, and many contemporary novelists claim to have developed their work entirely out of 'pictures in the mind' (Shepard, 1977).

Just as works of literature and scientific experiments can be prepared in the mind before being embodied, mental rehearsal of activity and its effects are well documented among athletes and other sports persons (Kiesler, 1984), who mentally 'run through' every part of a race or competition beforehand in order to overcome anxieties and self doubts and raise performance. Thus, the former athlete David Jenkins attributed his failure to add an Olympic gold medal to his many other sporting achievements to his inability to 'see' it happen. Olympic gold medalist David Hemery suggests that 'perhaps what is needed to achieve something more, something greater than ourselves, is to have vision beyond ourselves' (1978, p. 23). Indeed, imaginative procedures such as this are increasingly being advocated as necessary features of training by sports psychologists.

Rehearsal of images is also increasingly a feature of health psychology. Patients may be asked to imagine a malfunctioning organ as becoming normal. Clients in psychotherapy may be asked to practise imagining healthy interpersonal relationships, on the assumption that 'sane imagination will eventually lead to sane reality' (McMahon and Sheikh, 1984).

As Shepard indicates, these anecdotal reports

from various fields of endeavour do not establish that mental images actually played the crucial functional role attributed to them by scientists, authors and others. However, they nevertheless suggest that 'until we possess a more complete and satisfactory theory of the creative process, we run the risk of missing something of potential importance if we take it for granted that visual imagery is of no significance' (Shepard, 1977, p. 194).

Yet this is precisely the position adopted within psychology throughout the early years of the twentieth century, when imagery was relegated to 'the status of the nonexistent' by Watson, the founding father of behaviourism, who translated it into muscular contractions (Sheehan, 1972). Thus, although mental imagery had been one of the most important concepts for explaining and understanding human behaviour, it 'became suddenly a muted concern of the past' (Sheehan, 1972, p. xiii). All mental phenomena were identified with behaviour and psychologists went to great lengths to keep the term cognition out of their arguments. With the weakening of behaviourist strictures, imagery was acknowledged as a real and genuine subject for study but, as Sheehan indicates, 'such mentalistic sounding concepts were still relegated comfortably to the world of the poets'.

However, following the publication in 1964 of Holt's paper, *Imagery: the Return of the Ostracized* there was an increased interest in the topic. There was also a dramatic resurgence of interest after 1972, which Hearnshaw pinpoints as the year when cognitive psychology was reinstated as a legitimate area of investigation in psychology. Writing in that year Sheehan observed:

Far too many variables are now being manipulated systematically and related to imagery function for psychology to dismiss imagery as an unimportant construct for the explaining of higher mental functioning. Most recently, scientific psychology has been forced to look searchingly into its legitimate interests by having to account for the stunning effects of imagery as a mnemonic aid. Revitalizing some classical techniques of old, psychologists practising their science are demonstrating anew that people tutored in the use of imagery skills can perform at remarkable levels in comparison to those common to rote learning situations. Rather unfairly, imagery has had to prove itself worthy of notice by demonstrating more than ordinary effects before it could be rated equally with less exhibition-istic variables (Sheehan, 1972, p. xiii–xiv).

As he suggests, initially the application of mental imagery most commonly investigated was its use as a mnemonic or memory aid. It was established that one of the simplest ways of learning a list of items is to link the first and second items together as vividly as possible with a strong visual image and then produce a further image to link a third item and so on. This method of 'chaining' can be generalized to items other than words so that a sequence of ideas or actions can be memorized. Studies of the exceptional Russian mnemonist Shereshevskii in the 1920s by the psychologist Luria had established that he employed this method in his astonishing feats of memory. Typically he would remember a given list by summoning an image of its entirety, complete in its visual, auditory, tactile and even gustatory features. However, further investigation revealed that his efficiency could be increased further still by modification of this imagery such that one detail represented what formerly had been a whole scene. Simplified thus the image was less defined and vivid, but equally effective in aiding recall.

However, on deciding to become an entertainer, Shereshevskii began to use the visual image mnemonic known as the method of loci (from the Latin *locus* meaning place) in public performances. In this method a list or succession of ideas is committed to memory by imagining a familiar place and assigning images to certain landmarks or features of it. Typically, Shereshevskii would imagine himself walking down a familiar Moscow street, visualizing each item of a list in association with successive landmarks that he would then recall by mentally retracing his steps along the street. Hunter (1986) indicates that investigations of Shereshevskii failed to establish whether his ability for imagery was inborn or acquired, but clearly demonstrated that it could be brought under conscious control and put to intentional use. Subsequent research (Paivio, 1971, 1972) confirmed that non-verbal images can function as powerful mediators of memory and learning and are a critical component of meaning. His work reconciled imagery research with that on verbal learning, and it has since become clear that issues relating to memory, learning and information processing must all be considered in the context of visual imagery.

IMAGERY

Problem solving

Accounts by scientists and mathematicians of their use of imagery in the formulation and testing of hypotheses point not only to its potential application to problem solving but also to its superiority over language in certain situations. Within Western culture, with its emphasis on language skills, there is a tendency to represent issues verbally. This may be effective where issues lend themselves to verbal analysis, as Gellatly (1986) illustrates by reference to the following problem devised by the psychologist Edward de Bono.

You are organizing a singles knock-out tennis tournament for which there are 111 entrants. For each match there must be a new set of balls. How many sets of balls do you need to order?

It is difficult to imagine the draw for the tournament, and much easier to represent the problem verbally, as follows:

The number of entrants is 111. All of them lose once, except the winner of the tournament, so there must be 110 matches, and that is the number of boxes of balls required.

However verbal representation of some problems is not at all helpful, as Gellatly illustrates with reference to a problem devised by Duncker (1945).

One morning at sunrise, a Buddhist monk began to climb a mountain on a narrow path that wound around it. He climbed at a steady three miles per hour. After 12 hours he reached the top where there was a temple, and remained there to meditate for several days. Then, at sunrise, he started down the same path. He walked at a steady five miles per hour.

Prove that there must be a spot along the same path which he occupied on both trips at exactly the same time of day.

Here a visual representation of the problem as follows proves more efficient.

Imagine a monk climbing a mountain in the course of a day. Imagine also a second monk descending a mountain in the course of a day. Now super-impose the two images as if the two journeys were undertaken on the same day. Clearly at some point during the day the monks must meet and therefore be at the same point at the same time. This holds equally true for the case of a single monk making the two journeys on two separate days.

Verbal representation may not be particularly helpful in addressing issues, such as that above, which by their nature are non-verbal. In such cases, imagery provides an alternative means of representing such issues; a different way of looking at them, as it were, and in this mode novel features of which a person was formerly unaware or unconscious may become apparent. This is clearly not an either/or issue. In some cases the most efficient strategy is that which employs both kinds of representation. Hence flexibility of representation is desirable in effective problem solving.

Unfortunately, several factors tend to limit flexibility, and hence possibilities of problem solving in a given situation. These include mental habits acquired over the years that result in people becoming set in their ways and rigid in attitude and outlook. Negative thoughts, beliefs and expectations also greatly reduce the likelihood of new possibilities and solutions occurring. By allowing issues to be approached in a different way, and providing a new perspective on them, imagery may help to relax the rigid mental attitudes, beliefs, thoughts, expectations and habits that constrain people in inappropriate, ineffective, outmoded, and even unhealthy coping strategies, and introduce flexibility into cognitive functioning. In this sense, the alternative representation of issues afforded by imagery can 'shake up' or perturb existing mental patterns, enabling the person to 'see' solutions where formerly they could not, thereby bringing about transformation.

Individuals vary in the extent to which these factors influence their thinking, with the result that some are considerably more flexible in their representations than others. Nevertheless a major limiting factor in the attainment of flexibility of representation is the predominance of the verbal mode in Western culture, which ensures that for most people in the West the 'visionary mode' of representation is relatively less well developed. This is true also of Western psychology, which has emphasized the scientific study of language and verbal memory, and only very recently begun to investigate imaginal processes. Hence 'scientific study of mental imagery is a relatively recent development in psychology, even by the standards of the relatively young field of cognitive psychology' (Farah, 1989, p. 183). Moreover, it has been concerned almost exclusively with visual imagery and has largely neglected auditory, kinaesthetic and olfactory imagery.

The nature of mental imagery

Since the 1970s, research on mental imagery has focused on a number of closely related issues. These include whether mental imagery plays a significant functional role in human thinking, or whether it is merely a collection of epiphenomena which emerge when other memory and reasoning processes interact in particular ways, as has been suggested by Pylyshyn (1973, 1981) and what sort of physical processes underlie them in the brain.

Such questions are difficult to resolve empirically, or even clarify conceptually, because despite attempts to externalize them, mental images are inherently internal and subjective. Nevertheless, the development of non-introspective techniques for the study of imagery has not only shed significant light on these issues, but also stimulated further interest in this field of investigation.

The functional equivalence of imagery and visual perception

Roger Shepard (1977) argues that to the extent that mental images can substitute for perceptual images, subjects should be able to answer questions about objects as well when they are merely imagined as when directly perceived. Experiments carried out with various different objects have found no statistically significant difference between conditions in which various objects are physically presented or only imagined. Subjects base judgements only on identifiable physical properties of these objects (Shepard and Chipman, 1970; Shepard, 1975; Shepard and Cooper 1975; Shepard et al. 1975). These studies suggest that subjects perform very similar mental processes in the perceptual and imaginal conditions and that these processes operate on properties of the relevant objects, even when those objects are not physically present.

Shepard also argues that if perception and imagination use much of the same neural circuitry, then to imagine a particular object is to place oneself in a unique state of readiness for the actual perception of that particular object, and this should be revealed most sensitively in the reaction time to the corresponding test stimulus. Accordingly, he and his co-workers compared the time required to respond discriminatively to a test stimulus under conditions in which the subject has or has not already formed a preparatory visual image of the relevant stimulus. They found that once the relevant visual image has been formed, subjects are able to make the required discriminative response with great speed and accuracy. When no image, or an inappropriate image has been formed, subjects showed a consistent increase in reaction time. Consistent results were found with a variety of different sets of visual stimuli (Shepard and Metzler, 1971; Cooper and Shepard, 1973; Cooper, 1975), and supportive results have been obtained by other researchers (Shepard and Feng, 1972; Glusko and Cooper, 1978).

Cooper and Shepard (1973) also found that subjects respond to a test character in a rotated orientation with the same speed and accuracy when they prepare for the test by merely imagining the character in the appropriate orientation as when an actual outline of the character, already appropriately rotated, is physically presented to them. The finding that a purely mental image that is internally generated and transformed is virtually as effective as an external comparison stimulus already provided in that orientation is, they suggest, perhaps the most direct evidence available for a functional equivalence between imagery and perception.

These studies have only considered static images, yet scientists' self-reports suggest that it is possible to perform dynamic operations with images, and that it is this that confers on them most of their creative power. Tesla, Lawrence, Kekulé and Watson have all referred to rotations of images in space. Indeed, the notion of 'turning something over in one's mind' is quite commonplace. Like Helmholz (cited in Warren and Warren, 1969, pp. 252–4), it would seem that 'equipped with the awareness of the physical form of an object, we can clearly imagine all the perspective images which we may expect upon viewing from this or that side'.

Studies by Shepard and his co-researchers confirm that this is the case. They have found that under a broad range of conditions the time required to carry out an imagined operation in space increases, often in a remarkably linear manner, with the extent of the spatial transformation, for example, with angle in the case of rotation. This is equally true whether the mental operation is performed in the presence of the transformed physical object or in the imagination only. They interpret this as supporting the notion that mental transformation is carried out over a path that is the internal analogue of the corresponding physical transformation of the external object (Shepard and Metzler, 1971; Cooper and Shepard, 1973; Metzler and Shepard, 1974; Cooper, 1975).

Moreover, by measuring reaction times to variously oriented test stimuli presented during the course of mental rotation, they have established that the intermediate stages of the internal process have a one-to-one correspondence with intermediate orientations of the external object. Their results show there is actually something rotating during the course of a mental rotation, namely the orientation in which the corresponding external stimulus, if it were presented, would be most rapidly discriminated from other possible stimuli.

Shepard argues that the internal process that represents the transformations of an external object, just as much as the internal process that represents the object itself, is in large part the same, whether the transformation or the object is merely imagined or actually perceived. Accordingly, he proposes that imagery is an analogical or analogue process in which the internal states have a one-to-one correspondence to appropriate intermediate states in the external world. Thus, to imagine an object such as a complex molecule rotated in a different orientation is to perform an analogue process. Halfway through the process the internal state corresponds to the external object in an orientation halfway between the initial and final orientations. These analogue processes, he suggests, are particularly effective in dealing with complex structures and operations of such structures. Accordingly, he argues, by imagining various objects and their transformations in space one can explore many possibilities without taking the time, making the effort, or running the risk of carrying out those operations in physical reality.

Much recent research on mental imagery (a review of which is provided by Finke, 1989) focuses on the functional equivalence of imagery and visual perception, highlighting parallels between imagined and physical objects in respect to spatial arrangements of parts, dynamic characteristics and global organization. This appears to confirm Galton's assertion of almost a century ago that 'a visual image is the most perfect form of mental representation, wherever shape, position and relation of objects in space are concerned' (1883, p. 113).

Neuropsychological bases of imagery

The equivalence of imagery and visual perception has given rise to the belief that they activate similar physiological mechanisms. That is, images generate similar, albeit not necessarily identical internal response states as the actual stimuli themselves. The main source of supporting evidence comes from studies of brain-damaged patients with selective visual disorders and, more recently, from brain imaging techniques, some of which investigate regional brain activity during mental activity. However, as Farah (1989a) points out, little progress has been made in understanding the neurological basis of visual imagery.

Cognitive psychologists have largely avoided the latter in favour of attempting to understand mental imagery within an information processing paradigm.

She indicates that the most thoroughly studied of these imagery–perception parallels involves the phenomenon of visual neglect; that is, the failure of individuals to detect stimuli presented to half of the space opposite their brain lesion despite adequate elementary sensory processes. For example, patients with right parietal damage (those most likely to display neglect), may bump into people and objects on their left and leave food on the left side of their plate when still hungry, even though they are capable of seeing objects on the left if their attention is drawn to them. Several studies (Bisiach and Luzzatti, 1978; Bisiach, Luzatti and Persni, 1979; Bisiach et al., 1981; Ogden, 1985) have found that neglect of mental images accompanies visual neglect, and, according to Farah, constitute a strong demonstration that common mechanisms underlie imagery and perception. However, as she observes, it is difficult to be precise as to what component of imagery and perception is shared. Furthermore, it is possible to account for the common perceptual and imaginal deficit in terms of impaired attentional processes. Ogden (1985) provided some support for this idea, having found that all unilaterally brain-damaged patients, whether showing neglect in visual perception or not, and irrespective of the side of their lesions, neglected the contra-lesional side of their images. However, further evidence in support of the premise that nonsensory visual structures that normally subserve object recognition are also involved in object imagery, has been provided (Shuttleworth, Syring and Allen, 1982; Farah, 1984; Levine, Warach and Farah, 1985).

Brain imaging techniques with normal subjects, which use a variety of indices of regional cerebral activity, such as electrical activity, metabolic activity or blood flow, offer far greater spatial precision than the effects of naturally occurring brain damage for the functional isolation and anatomical localization of cognitive systems. Farah (1989a) reports a number of studies using these techniques which have revealed activation during mental imagery in sensory regions of the visual system. She indicates that various studies employing electrophysiological techniques (EEG, electroencephalography; and ERP, event-related potentials) have also provided evidence that mental imagery evokes visual sensory activity in normal subjects. Farah therefore concludes:

> measures of regional cerebral blood flow and electrical activity have demonstrated visual cortex involvement in imagery, including the involvement of regions classically considered to be sensory processing areas. Other evidence, from studies of focally brain-damaged patients, highlight some of the nonsensory components of vision that are shared with mental imagery. On the one hand, these results support the old and intuitively appealing idea, first expressed by Hume, that mental images are reactivations of perceptual experiences. On the other hand, they count as strong disconfirming evidence against the current view of some cogni-

tive psychologists that mental images are abstract, propositional memory representations unrelated to perception (1989a, p. 190).

Indeed, Farah (1984) claims that the results of her study of visual deficit support the existence of an imagery system distinct from other memory and reasoning processes, with an internal structure corresponding to components outlined by Kosslyn (1980) and later expanded by herself.

Components of visual imagery

Kosslyn proposed a structure, which he termed the visual buffer, as the medium in which images occur, claiming that the spatial/pictorial information-bearing structure consciously experienced as an image, consists of patterns of activation in the visual buffer that generate, inspect and transform the image. The generation process creates the image in the visual buffer from information stored in long-term visual memory. The inspection process converts the patterns of activation in the visual buffer into organized percepts by identifying parts and relations within the image, and the transformation processes rotate and translate it.

To Kosslyn's model, Farah has added: a descriptive component for question-answering tasks in which the contents of the visual buffer can be inspected and described; a copy component for constructional tasks in which the contents of the visual buffer must be inspected and drawn or constructed; a detection component for simple visual perception tasks and introspective imagery tasks in which the patterns of activation in the visual buffer need not be processed but the mere presence of activation must be detected; and a recognition process by which responses derived from the input and long-term visual memories are matched.

Pylyshyn (1981) has claimed, that imagery consists of recalling and manipulating information about the appearances of objects in a way that is not fundamentally different from other memory contents such as historical facts. Farah argues that if this were the case, one would not expect to find cases of selective loss of imagery ability any more than of selective loss of history ability, and one would certainly not expect to find a separate brain area dedicated to one of these abilities. Yet her findings are suggestive of a consistent pattern of deficit in the reports of patients with loss of mental imagery following brain damage, which could be attributed to the image generation component of imagery, and which implicate a region in the posterior left hemisphere of the brain as critical for the image generation process. Furthermore, her analysis of the neurological literature on loss of mental imagery suggests that the long-term memories used in imagery are also used in object recognition, and that dreaming and waking imagery share some underlying processes. On this basis she concludes that imagery shares representations with perceptual processes in the brain, a conclusion supported by Heil, Roster and Hennghausen (1993), who suggest that there is definite interaction between imagery and perceptual processes.

The implications of this analysis for understanding intact imagery system in normal humans are, as Farah indicates, considerable. They suggest there is neuropsychological evidence for the existence of an image generation process, distinct from long-term visual memories themselves and other recall processes, and a functional localization for that process. Moreover, the specific location indicated for image generation calls into question widely held assumptions about the neurological bases of imagery.

Neurological bases of imagery

Greater understanding of brain function has resulted from the so-called 'split-brain' research initiated by Roger Sperry (1962, 1966). This arose, and gained its name, from attempts to confine severe epileptic seizures to one hemisphere of the brain by surgically cutting the connective tissue between the two halves of the cortex. In such cases neural transmission is severed, and what might be thought of as communication between the two sides of the brain is cut off.

Although this surgery proved effective in restricting the severity of epilepsy, it was found to have other rather less desirable consequences, notably that the patients effectively had two independent brains controlling their bodies, often with bizarre consequences. As a result, their left hand did not know what the right hand was doing, quite literally. Personality and emotion were also adversely affected, as Sperry and his co-workers vividly illustrated. These outcomes served to highlight the different cognitive functions of the left and right hemispheres. As a result of these initial experiments a firm association was established between the left hemisphere and verbal/linguistic processes, and between the right hemisphere and visual/spatial cognitive processes.

These findings were brought to wide public attention by Ornstein (1972), who, in addition to describing the cognitive properties of each hemisphere, also ascribed different modes of consciousness to them. He asserted that these had evolved from the analytic *versus* holistic cognitive styles of the left and right hemispheres, respectively.

Using cerebral laterality as a metaphor for personal cognitive styles, Ornstein implied that a strong tendency existed for individuals to use preponderantly one hemisphere or the other to experience the world and to cognize the information in it. Thus people could be classified according to their 'hemisphericity'. The notion of individual hemisphericity was extrapolated to groups of individuals: it was suggested that different cultures were more prone to rely on either a left- or right-hemisphere mode of information processing. In short, Ornstein differentiated Eastern and Western modes of experience and related these to hemispheric differences in cognitive style (Ley and Smylie, 1989, p. 326).

Subsequently, as Ley and Smylie point out, the scientific study of brain laterality became a psychological zeitgeist, yielding a tenfold increase in research articles in this domain between 1970 and 1980. This research initially appeared to confirm that the two cerebral hemispheres are specialized for different cognitive functions. The left hemisphere being primarily concerned with language and language-related functions, and the right hemisphere with a variety of nonlinguistic visual/spatial functions (Ornstein *et al.*, 1979; Ley and Bryden, 1983), mental imaging (Ley, 1983) and emotion (Tucker *et al.*, 1977; Ley and Bryden, 1983).

Right hemispheric localization of image generation

Various loci in the right hemisphere have been suggested as concerned with imagery, including the parietal, occipital and temporal lobes. Achterberg (1985) identifies pre-frontal lobes or most anterior aspects of the frontal lobes as a possible site. She indicates that although the function of these areas remains uncertain they appear to be involved in memory storage and emotion. They also have connections with the limbic system, that area of the brain which processes emotion, so numerous that the anterior and frontal lobes appear to be an extension of the emotional system itself. Studies have suggested that this area is necessary for immediate memory or use by symbolic memory images (Jacobsen, 1936), and that damage to the right frontal lobe affects image storage and retrieval (Milner, 1971). Frontal lobotomy patients have been found not only to lack emotion but to be unable to hold symbolic imagery (Meyer and Beck, 1954). A study by Humphrey and Zangwill (1951), of patients with damage to posterior parietal areas of the right hemisphere, found little or no dreaming, dim waking imagery and an inability to function in tasks requiring visual, olfactory and auditory phenomena. This is frequently cited as providing evidence for the involvement of other right hemispheric lobes in imagery. Achterberg (1985) cites other studies as furnishing further evidence to this effect. More recently Bisiach and Berti (cited Sheikh, Kunzendorf and Sheikh, 1989) have suggested that the right posterior cortical structures are especially crucial to conscious visual imagery.

A psychosomatic model of brain function

Achterberg (1985) has drawn on the well-established assumption that the right hemisphere is primarily implicated in imagery and emotion, and activated during stress, in proposing a neuroanatomic model of image function in the mediation of brain and bodily processes. However, as she indicates (Achterberg, 1985, p. 126), 'other areas of the brain besides the cortical hemispheres are obviously necessary to move consciousness downward to contact and alter physiology'. She argues that if the right hemisphere is primarily implicated in emotion it must have a direct relationship with the autonomic nervous system. She supports this supposition by pointing to the vast network of neural connections between the right hemisphere and the limbic system, which she identifies as a processing area for the emotions, the activities of which involve the autonomic nervous system. She also points to a structural and functional relations between the limbic system, which she describes as 'the outcropping of the image-laden frontal lobes' (p. 126) and the hypothalamus (which regulates body rhythms, heart rate, respiration, blood chemistry, glandular activity and immune functions) and between the hypothalamus and the pituitary gland (which regulates the hormonal systems of the body, affecting every organ, tissue and cell of the body). Achterberg claims that there is sufficient evidence about the specific functions of the right hemisphere, and its connections with other brain and body components, to support the premise that images 'can and do carry information from the conscious fore to the far reaches of the cells' (Achterberg, 1985, p. 122). In this way they mediate between mental and bodily processes: 'The evidence for the neuroanatomical bridge between image and cells, mind and body, exists. It is solid, and can be viewed when brain tissue is placed under a microscope' (Achterberg, 1985, p. 127).

Achterberg suggests that because the verbal functions of the left hemisphere are one step removed from the autonomic processes, both in evolution and function, messages have to undergo transformation by the right hemisphere into non-verbal or imagerial terminology before they can be understood by the involuntary or autonomic nervous system. Similarly, before the imagery characteristic of right hemispheric functions can be processed into meaningful logical thought it must be translated by the left hemisphere. The images intimately connected with physiology, health and disease are, she argues, preverbal, without a language base, except what is available through connections with the left hemisphere. If these connections were to be severed and the left hemisphere thereby rendered inaccessible, untranslated messages would continue to affect emotions and alter physiology, but without intellectual interpretation. She points to the disorder alexithymia (literally, without words for feelings) as suggesting that this does occur. In this, as yet little understood, condition emotions and images which remain untranslated are thought to be expressed physically in various body systems, and the resulting damage eventually diagnosed as rheumatoid arthritis, ulcerative colitis, asthma, hives, migraine and other psychosomatic disorders.

By virtue of linguistic communication with others the left hemisphere may be conceptualized as an interface with the external world. Accordingly, Achterberg proposes that the imagery of the right hemisphere is the medium of communication between consciousness and the inner world of the body, serving as the means whereby 'unconscious' non-verbal physiological processes become conscious or verbalizable. The limbic system is the area in which this 'translation' occurs. Moreover, as is the case with any bridge or 'border' area (from the Latin *limbus* meaning border), it can, in principle at least, be used in two directions, and therefore translate verbal messages into non-verbal imagerial terminology. Imagery is therefore construed as a bridge not only between left and right hemispheric processes but also between different levels of the self; between psyche and soma. As such, Achterberg claims a role in psychology for imagination similar to that conceived by Aristotle, in whose cognitive psychology it was the bridge between sensation and thought: 'Imagination is impossible without sensation, and conceptual thought is impossible without imagination' (extract from *De Memoria* cited Hearnshaw, 1989, p. 25).

In the context of imaginative medicine the notion of images as transformers or translators of different kinds of 'message' or information in the brain is in itself quite persuasive. It accounts quite adequately for both the physiological effects of imagery and its diagnostic reliability. Furthermore, the limbic system would appear to be a probable location for such processes (see Chapter 3). However, the neuropsychological links between imagery, emotion and immune functioning are not as clear cut as Achterberg suggests. Indeed, as Paivio (1989) observes, the complexity of the problem is evident in the diversity of views concerning the cerebral localization of imagery.

Left hemispheric localization of image generation

Although the most common and longstanding view, supported by considerable evidence (Ley, 1983) is that imagery is predominantly a right hemisphere function, it now seems clear that neither hemisphere can be excluded. Indeed, the assumption made by numerous authors that imagery is a right hemispheric function is not supported by the available evidence. A left parietal basis for imagery was first proposed in 1947. Erhlichman and Barrett (1983) claim that although Humphrey and Zangwill's (1951) study is often cited in support of a right hemisphere locus for imagery, the authors themselves asserted that 'disorders of visual imagination appear liable to follow lesions on either side'. More recent studies (Farah, 1984; Kosslyn *et al.*, 1985) have indicated that the left hemisphere predominates in image generation, albeit not necessarily in other image functions. An analysis by Farah (1984) of relevant neuropsychological research, points to the possibility that the critical area for image generation may be close to posterior language centres of the left hemisphere. She has since pointed to a number of other studies, where 'in each case, the lesion was in the distribution of the left posterior cerebral artery, and affected mainly the occipito–temporal regions of the left hemisphere' (Farah, 1989a, p. 192). She observes,

> Whatever the precise intrahemispheric localization of image generation, one of the most interesting aspects of the results...is that they seem to suggest that image generation is a lateralized function of the brain. Furthermore, these results contradict the widely held assumption, first explicitly noted by Ehrlichman and Barrett (1983), that imagery processes are carried out in the right hemisphere (Farah, 1989a, p. 192).

The results of a further study that attempted to test the hypothesis of left hemisphere specialization for image generation in normal subjects (Farah, 1986), are consistent with a left hemisphere basis for image generation. However, they suggest that the left hemisphere is relatively more adept at image generation than the right, in contradistinction to an earlier study (Farah *et al.*,

1985) that suggested an absolute rather than a relative, left hemisphere specialization for image generation.

Many other neuropsychological studies have found evidence of left hemisphere involvement in image generation, although in most cases the these studies were not undertaken with this hypothesis in mind. In many cases, the results of these studies were discounted by the original investigators as representing the involvement of (or contamination by) language or 'analytic' strategies in their imagery tasks. However, there appears to be no strong reason to interpret these findings thus, except for the *a priori* belief that imagery is not a left hemisphere function (compare Erhlichman and Barrett, 1983) and the knowledge that language is (Farah, 1989a, p. 195).

However, the issue is by no means resolved. Whereas the studies reviewed by Farah could indicate damage to the non-verbal representation systems necessary for image generation they could also indicate damage to the referential connections between language and image systems because the imagery deficits are largely inferred from the inability of subjects to generate images to verbal cues. Paivio (1989) concludes that the evidence indicates left hemisphere dominance in tasks that require referential processing. These include tasks in which mental images must be generated in words or described verbally, although he acknowledges that some degree of language-evoked imagery is possible in the right hemisphere. He therefore presents another interpretation, namely that both hemispheres 'contain' the information and mechanisms required for experiencing and using imagery. He claims that such a view has been supported empirically by Bisiach *et al.* (1981).

These findings on image generation are consistent with the results of other studies on brain lateralization during the 1980s. These prompted an awareness that the findings of earlier studies should not be taken to mean that a particular hemisphere has sole responsibility for a particular cognitive task, and that the differences should be regarded as relative rather than absolute, even for well-lateralized functions. Thus, although the left brain has executive control of language and language-related functions, the right hemisphere has a rudimentary language capacity. Indeed, while the left is responsible for processing the phonological, syntactic and semantic aspects of language (Segalowitz, 1983), the right is concerned with processing information related to highly emotional or imageable words (Bryden and Ley, 1983).

Other well-established notions about cerebral laterality, such as the links between the right hemisphere and emotional processes, have also been challenged (Silberman and Weingartner, 1986). This research suggests that the left hemisphere is involved in the processing of positive emotions and in the stimulation of the immune system. The right hemisphere is involved in the processing of negative emotions and in the suppression of the nervous system, either directly or by mediating and/or inhibiting the activity of the left. This finds some support in the observations of Geschwind and Behan (1982). They reported that left-handed people are more susceptible to auto-immune disorders.

Others (Wechsler, 1987, cited by Pelletier and Herzing, 1989) have suggested that patients who exercise the right hemisphere during imagery exercises may 'distract' it from suppressing the immune system. They claim that 'comprehending these neurophysiological mechanisms of cognitive activation and control will be critical to understanding immunological competence' (Pelletier and Herzing, 1989, p. 371).

Ley and Smylie (1989) conclude that despite research findings linking specific functions to each hemisphere, such differences relate more to the 'style' of information processing than the information that is being processed. 'In other words, it is not so much the case that each hemisphere is uniquely specialized to work with different 'things' (e.g. the left hemisphere with phonemes and the right hemisphere with musical tones), rather, it is that each hemisphere is organized structurally to provide a different cognitive style. Each style is more or less well adapted to processing different types of information' (Ley and Smylie, 1989, p. 330). Sergent (1982) has also challenged characterization of the left hemisphere as a logical, analytical and sequential processor, and the right hemisphere as a holistic and diffuse processor. He argues that the left hemisphere is best suited for 'detailed' processing that can be most aptly considered as 'high-resolution' or 'high-frequency' information, and the right hemisphere better suited to processing larger non-detailed 'low frequency' information.

However, reviewing the available evidence, Paivio (1989) concludes that all the suggestions emerging from the research are partly correct, 'Neural structures in both hemispheres must have the representational information and processing capacities associated with imagery phenomena, but they participate differentially in different functions of imagery' (p. 203). In his view, therefore, imagery is multifaceted and not localized in any specific brain area; different regions in both cerebral hemispheres, and possibly also subcortical regions, being responsible for different imagery functions. He identifies the posterior regions of both hemispheres as appearing to contain the representational information necessary for the activation and generation of images of objects. He suggests that both may be equally efficient in such semantic memory tasks as symbolic size comparison of objects, whereas the left hemisphere may dominate when the task simply requires referential imagery, for example generation of unitary images to verbal cues, or when images must be described. However, the left hemisphere might not be so favoured if images are generated associatively to non-verbal cues. He identifies posterior regions of the right hemisphere as crucial in non-verbal spatial organizational and transformational functions involving imagery, and suggests that the right hemisphere might also dominate in emotional and memory functions of imagery. More specifically, he proposes the right temporal lobe as the possible focal region for storage or retrieval of episodic memory images, or as a crucial mediator of such functions in other areas.

Therapeutic functions of imagery

The precise neurophysiological and neuropsychological mechanisms underlying imagery are still far from understood. However, it seems that the key to understanding its function lies in its role as a transformer or transducer of information in the brain. It facilitates the translation of both verbal and non-verbal outputs and 'communication' between relevant processes. Contemporary research supports the age-old wisdom that images effect a link between cognition and sensation (mind and body) and thus between essentially conscious processes amenable to language and those that are not. Such images provide an insight into the more 'primitive' mind of man.

As an alternative, albeit complementary cognitive representational mode to the verbal, imagery provides, quite literally a new perspective on, or way of looking at issues. It is therefore particularly suited to the representation of issues which in themselves are non-verbal. For example, physiological and emotional processes, that are relevant to both physical and psychological health. By so doing it increases the range and flexibility of mental functioning, providing a tool which greatly benefits problem solving, decision making and creative thinking. As imagery and perception are neurologically similar processes, experience in the imagination can be viewed as psychologically equivalent to actual experience. Thus, as a means of 'reality' testing and problem solving it is often superior to 'rational' logical strategies. Moreover, because imagery is isomorphic with perception it has a greater capacity for descriptive accuracy than verbal logic which is linear rather than a simultaneous representation (Sheikh and Panagiotou, 1975). Houston (1982, p. 135) in describing this 'patterning of ideas and images gathered up in a simultaneous constellation' points to the fact that thinking in images is very much quicker than verbal thinking. It is instantaneous and global rather than sequential, and, in the manner of visual perception, conveys complex information more immediately than verbal language. Therefore, as Shepard (1977) indicates, possibilities can be explored in the imagination without taking the time, making the effort or running the risk of carrying out those operations in physical reality.

The simultaneous representation of images results in a time sense or perception of time quite unrelated to serial clock time. This effectively relieves pressures and tensions associated with time-related stress. Together with the absorbing quality of imagery, it promotes relaxation, thereby increasing the flexibility of functioning (both mental and physical) and awareness, the two key characteristics of healthy functioning and survival.

Images relate to physiological states in ways suggesting both a causative and reactive role (Achterberg, 1985). Therefore the physiological effects produced by imagery can be induced consciously and deliberately or unconsciously. Imagery can also provide important clues as to physiological functioning. It therefore provides a tool for accessing and utilizing mental and physiological processes of which people are generally unaware or unconscious, and as such is an important tool for self-discovery and creative change. Panagiotou and Sheikh (1977) suggest that imagery may be a more direct expression of the unconscious than linguistic expression. It is less likely to be filtered through the conscious critical apparatus, because generally words and phrases must be consciously understood before they are spoken; that is, they must pass through a rational censorship before they can assume grammatical order. In the light of the foregoing characteristics of imagery, Sheikh, Kunzendorf and Sheikh (1989, p. 493) therefore conclude:

> It seems reasonable to believe that images hold enormous potential for healing, and it is not surprising that extensive claims about the promise of imagery for therapeutic benefits have been made. A large body of recent scientific research on imagery indicates that these claims are justified. However, direct systematic research on the therapeutic outcome of imagery approaches with clients suffering from a variety of ailments is urgently needed.

5

Translating theory into practice

Knowing how an egg boils is not the same as knowing how to boil one.
Phil Hogan

Sheikh, Kunzendorf and Sheikh (1989) note that 'in the last two decades, imagery has risen from a position of near disgrace to become one of the hottest topics in both clinical and experimental cognitive psychology' (p. 489). Research has largely focused attention on the cognitive function of imagery in affording an alternative means of mental representation. It has highlighted the usefulness of imagery in facilitating problem solving, decision making, creative thinking and improved coping strategies. Greater understanding of the functions of imagery has led to its application in various fields.

GENERAL USES OF IMAGERY

Increasingly, imagery is being used in training decision making and problem solving skills by business and management consultants, and in stimulating creative thinking (Morgan, 1993). It is also being used as an aid to relaxation and improved coping skills by stress management consultants, and in assertiveness training. Teachers are beginning to use imagery for similar purposes. The tension-reducing features of imagery can be applied to assist in classroom control and to help students cope with potentially stressful situations, such as examinations. Imagery is also being used as a tool for accessing issues which may be difficult for individuals, especially children, to articulate, such as abuse and bullying, emotional and physical pain (Oaklander, 1978; Roet, 1988; Jackson, 1993). These methods are increasingly being used in social work. Imagery techniques are also being exploited in the commercial field. In advertising, they are used to explore unconscious associations to advertised products, including medicines. In public relations, subjects' responses to public figures, such as politicians, are used as the basis for impression management and image building (Branthwaite and Cooper, 1989).

THERAPEUTIC USES OF IMAGERY

Imagery is most widely used within the health-care and related professions where its therapeutic benefits are increasingly being recognized and supported by research. Apart from any physiological changes they might effect, the processes of the imagination are widely acknowledged as potent therapeutic agents.

Researchers have ascribed the clinical efficacy of images to a variety of processes, both cognitive and emotional (Sheikh, Kunzendorf and Sheikh, 1989). These include: the client's clear discrimination of his or her ongoing fantasy processes; the clues regarding alternative approaches to various situations afforded by images; awareness of usually avoided situations; the opportunity images provide for covert rehearsal of alternate approaches; consequent decrease in fear of overtly approaching avoided situations (Singer, 1974); and the feeling of control and enhanced coping skills gained from monitoring and rehearsing various images (Meichenbaum, 1978; Sheikh and Jordan, 1983). Images are also a source of detail about past experiences (Sheikh and Panagiotou, 1975), providing access to significant memories of early childhood before language became predominant (Kepecs, 1954), and other features of which a person is largely unconscious (Panagiotou and Sheikh, 1977). They afford a richer experience of a range of emotions (Singer, 1979); are effective in by-passing defences and resistances (Klinger, 1971; Reyher, 1963; Singer, 1974); and frequently open up new avenues for exploration when therapy reaches an impasse (Sheikh and Jordan, 1983).

Clinicians generally prefer to work with a person's spontaneously generated imagery. However, where a person's representation of issues is too limited to enable coping in a given area, or where a therapist wishes to challenge existing representations, guided imagery techniques are frequently used. Indeed the therapeutic effectiveness of these methods has been attributed to two major functions: the opportunity they provide to present a person with an experience which is the basis for representation of issues in his or her cognitive model where previously there has been little or none; and to challenge the person's presently impoverished model (Bandler and Grinder, 1975). Thus, although it is preferable to work with a person's spontaneous imagery where possible, recognition of the effectiveness of guided imagery in introducing greater flexibility of cognitive functioning has led to its proliferation within psychotherapy and counselling. Similarly, guided imagery is being applied as an adjunct to orthodox medical approaches in helping individuals and their families to cope with a wide range of illnesses and medical treatments, including radiotherapy, chemotherapy and surgery; and related issues such as pain, death, bereavement, social isolation, trauma and disability.

GUIDED IMAGERY AS MEDICINE

Certainly, over the past 20 years or so 'Experimental and clinical psychologists have...produced a considerable body of literature documenting that images are indeed a powerful force' (Sheikh, Kunzendorf and Sheikh, 1989, p. 489); with both psychological and physical effects. Dossey (1982) has claimed that the effects associated with imagery are as potent and real as those produced by any drug, and, accordingly, that imagery should be regarded as medicine in the truest sense of the word. Arguably, therefore, imagery techniques should be subject to similar controls in relation to testing, administration, advertising and the claims made for them. Yet this is clearly not the case, as is most evident in the recent enthusiastic promotion and popularization of guided therapy techniques as a means of self-help therapy.

Variously referred to as creative visualization, creative imagination and guided fantasy, these techniques are often collectively and misleadingly termed visualization therapy. This implies that mental imagery is necessarily visual, which is not the case. Imagery may involve any of the senses, or a combination of them. As a mental representation it involves not merely 'seeing' a picture in the mind's eye but sensing or experiencing it in various ways. The term also implies that simply forming mental images is therapeutic, rather than the healing process they may facilitate. However, imagery can and does produce non-therapeutic effects in much the same way as any drug. Thus, while it is fair to claim images are therapeutic, to the extent that they can facilitate and enhance relaxation, it is nevertheless true that their effects can be quite the opposite, as in the case of hallucinations, nightmares, 'flashback' experiences and phobias. Indeed the therapeutic value of imagery lies not in the images themselves but in what they may reveal about physical, psychological and spiritual aspects of personal functioning, and the possibilities these insights afford for creative change and self-development. Therefore, like any drug, psychological or medical treatment, the therapeutic value of imagery depends on how it is used.

Three major factors influence the way in which any treatment, including imagery, is used, and determine its effectiveness: the treatment itself; the therapist who prescribes and/or administers the treatment; and the person who receives it. Commonly, it is assumed that the therapist and the recipient are different people. Yet most people treat themselves, initially at least, irrespective of their condition, and may continue to do so even when they receive treatment from others. This often overlooked factor is taken into account in the following discussion which, in an attempt to avoid confusion uses the term 'guide' to refer to anyone, professional or lay, who uses imagery as a form of self-help therapy or instructs others in its use, whether in books or by way of other media, or directly on a one-to-one or group basis.

Packaging treatment

The 'packaging' of a therapy (the way it is presented to the public) may be as or more important than the nature of the therapy itself. Placebo effects are achieved, seemingly, by the ability of a substance or procedure to seize the imagination and to please. It is on this basis, very frequently, that a therapy is sold to consumers, be they medical practitioners or patients. Drug companies go to considerable lengths to establish the image associated in the public mind with their products (Branthwaite and Cooper, 1989). Similarly, guided imagery techniques, the specific aim of which is to capture the imagination so as to use its effects directly, are attractively packaged for the public at large. This may reflect popular trends and fashions, topical concerns, creative thinking, decision making, stress management, coping skills, lifestyle change, health, healing, personal development or spiritual growth. In being 'shaped' to conform in these ways the impressions given may be misleading.

Claims made for guided imagery

As has been noted, the claims made for imagery are impressive, and research supports the potency of imagery in a range of applications. However, the claims are sometimes exaggerated, especially in relation to health and healing, where guided imagery is often promoted as a cure for all ills. Reports in the medical and psychological literature concerning its beneficial effects as adjuvant therapy in the treatment of cancers and other serious illnesses have led to claims that imagery is a cure for cancer. Some individuals have advocated rejection of conventional medical treatment for cancer and AIDS in favour of guided imagery techniques and lifestyle changes (Brohn, 1986; Asistent and Duffy, 1991). However, Ornstein and Sobel (1988) indicate that although there have been many claims for the effects of imagery on diseases there is little convincing scientific evidence that alone it can cure serious illness.

Pelletier and Herzing (1989) indicate that although improved cancer outcomes have been reported in response to guided imagery, relaxation and hypnotic induction, immunosuppression by way of psychological factors is much more frequently reported in the research literature than immunoenhancement. Indeed, this latter phenomenon remains controversial as it is by no means clear whether it exists. Pelletier and Herzing (1989, p. 356) indicate that while it may be possible to enhance immunological responses above baseline, there are several alternative possibilities which might account for this apparent effect. These extremely complex issues are far from resolution. Enhancement may simply be restoration of normal baseline functions. Selective suppression of cells in the immune system may produce the illusion that others are enhanced. There may be a rebound effect in which a stressor temporarily suppresses an immune marker, which then rebounds to an apparent higher value when the stressor ceases. Moreover, as they indicate, the clinical significance of immunological variability is unknown, and there is no empirical basis to determine the magnitude of immunological impairment necessary to be causally linked to increased disease susceptibility, onset or intervention. Accordingly, there is a need for greater caution in the claims made for the beneficial effects of imagery on immune functions and disease.

It is also important to establish that the imagery procedures recommended are appropriate to a person's needs, and have some proven utility in this regard. As a general principle it is accepted that the claims made for drugs in advertising have been subject to rigorous testing, not only to establish that observable effects are the results of the drug rather than the imagination, but also to establish any contraindications to their use. Drug trials are therefore held to be a standard procedure, although this represents the ideal rather than actual practice. However, no such ideal exists in regard to imaginative medicine, much less in practice. Imagery exercises are therefore generally untested and of dubious validity and reliability, either as a tool for phenomenological investigation and research or as a therapeutic procedure.

The formulae of many guided imagery exercises are literally dreamt up by therapists and authors on the basis of personal symbolism, or concocted piecemeal from archetypal symbols culled from various sources, on the assumption that because these elements have proved personally meaningful and valuable they will be likewise for others. This implicit theory is almost never put to any kind of empirical test, with the result that the validity and reliability of the exercises in addressing, much less effecting certain issues, remain open to question. Results obtained from small, discrete samples of subjects may also be unreliable when generalized to an entire population, as early studies in the application of imagery techniques in the treatment of cancer revealed.

In their initial treatment programme the Simontons asked cancer patients (all US Air Force servicemen) to imagine their cancer being destroyed and disposed of by their body's immune system. They noted that those patients who succeeded in overcoming their cancer usually employed imagery with certain qualitative features: the cancer cells were represented as weak, confused and susceptible to breakdown and the treatment as strong and powerful. The body's immune system was imagined as an aggressive army of white blood cells, eager to do battle with invading organisms and destroy them. Dead cancer cells were then imagined being removed from the body normally and naturally, leaving it free of cancer and healthy, and the person able to reach his or her goals in life. The Simontons therefore identified imagery which matched these criteria as essentially positive, and advocated their use by patients attempting to overcome cancer. Such imagery has since been widely adopted by cancer patients, as is highlighted in 11-year-old Joanne Gillespie's account of her fight against cancer:

> I visualize cancer cells as grey weak soldiers and my good cells as a
> strong white army of good fighters. I make the two armies fight and see

all the grey soldiers smashed up and killed – no prisoners my Mam and Dad say – and I always make sure of that. Then a big waterfall runs right through my body washing away all the dead soldiers. I do this listening to music, sometimes soft music with no words. Then I visualize myself as I want to be – strong healthy and dancing.

CRITERIA FOR GUIDED IMAGERY

In association with the Simontons, Achterberg and Lawlis (1978) drew up a list of tentative criteria for assessing the imagery of cancer patients. They observe that representations of cancer cells as ants, or eggs in an incubator, are essentially negative, suggesting the likely proliferation of the disease. Similarly, they suggest that images of crabs and other crustaceans which are tenacious and have hard impregnable shells symbolize the potency of the disease. They also point out that imagery may betray negative expectancies about treatment. For example, imagery where chemotherapy is imagined as yellow pills being greedily consumed by a large black rat symbolizing the cancer, portrays the latter as strong and invasive and treatment as weak and impotent. They argue that it is especially important in treating malignancy that the most powerful imagery relates to the person's own natural defence system, rather than the disease or treatment. They propose that the individual should be encouraged to imagine the white blood cells of the body at least as vividly as the malignant cells, but as more numerous and powerful. The individual must also achieve powerful images of the latter being removed from the body. In addition, treatment should be imagined as a friend or ally, and patients encouraged to personalize it in any way that seems appropriate. This, they suggest, helps to reduce the aversive side-effects of treatment, and, as has been reported subsequently, there is some evidence to support this claim.

Simonton and Simonton (1975) indicate, however, that while those who succeed in overcoming cancer generally have, or achieve imagery that matches these criteria, it does not necessarily contain all these elements at the outset. Imagery needs to be guided, to enable the patient to discover sufficiently powerful images to capture a new positive expectation. They recognize that mental imagery involves a highly personal symbolic language, and that the emotional meaning of any one symbol will vary greatly from one person to another. Thus one person's image of strength and power may signify weakness to another. Given such variation the importance of exploring personal imagery with an individual rather than imposing meaning on it is emphasized. The meaning of this personal imagery may not be readily apparent to the individual, and so in order to translate its inherent beliefs and expectations and discover its meaning it may be necessary for the person to 'try on' the image. Simonton and Simonton therefore advocate free drawing and other means of exploring imagery as valuable methods for facilitating discussion and understanding.

Given the need for vivid and powerful imagery, they recommend that the white cells are imagined as dogs voraciously eating minced meat (the cancer) and licking the area clean. In so doing, it would seem that they fall into the very trap they advise others against, inasmuch as they are not only imposing their imagery rather than encouraging people to generate their own, but also suggesting imagery of a curiously ambiguous nature. Whereas to some people dogs may be 'man's best friend', those who are not dog lovers, or have been bitten by a dog, may fear that such 'voracious' animals might not be satisfied with minced meat and 'turn' on them.

Indeed, a good deal of the imagery recommended by the Simontons (Simonton and Simonton, 1975) may provoke ambivalent responses. Current thinking is that the early work on the use of the imagination in the treatment of cancer placed too much emphasis on anger, killing and hating, and that as a result some people were repelled by it. It seems that because the initial patient group were members of the armed forces and were not squeamish about attacking and killing cancer cells, they assumed that everyone would be equally comfortable with these notions. In fact, as Siegel (1986) observes, many people are profoundly disturbed by the idea of attacking and killing anything, even an invading disease organism. Words (much favoured by the medical profession) such as assault, kill, insult, blast, poison and destroy, might therefore be rejected either consciously or unconsciously by some people. Left to summon their own imagery people may very well devise equally effective but more gentle means of dealing with and disposing of their disease. Arguably, in the case of cancer, such an approach is more appropriate because it is the body's own cells which have gone awry, and, in a sense, a direct aggressive attack on them constitutes an attack on the self.

There are other reasons why gentler images may be more appropriate. Although the immune system is commonly viewed as the body's defence system, designed to seek out and destroy harmful and alien substances, such as bacteria and viruses, it is now recognized as functioning with more subtlety than this warlike metaphor suggests (Taylor, 1990). Indeed, what has been described as the 'battlefield' terminology of immunology has had to be reappraised in the light of evidence which suggests that, rather than being in any sense combative, the immune system operates co-operatively and collaboratively to support the integrity of the body and its optimal relationship to its environment. From this perspective, disease can more appropriately be viewed as disharmony or lack of coherence rather than an unnatural disease entity or state that needs to be fought. Taylor observes, therefore, that while classically the immune system has been seen in terms of soldiery defending the body against invaders, more recent appreciation of the subtlety of its activities suggests that a better metaphor might be that of a gardener.

Nevertheless, Manning (1988, 1989) emphasizes the importance of 'fighting' imagery. He argues that people who resist aggressive imagery often confuse anger with assertiveness, and that if such a person is angry and his or her imagery is passive then the anger has no release, whereas imagery that is initially aggressive becomes progressively less so as the anger is released. He also observes that a person is more powerful when angry than when passive and that this strength may be mobilized in support of healing. Support for Manning's observations is provided by research which has linked inability to express anger with cancer. Significantly better treatment outcomes have also been noted in patients who can express their anger compared with those who cannot. Recent awareness within the scientific community suggests that cancer may be caused by failure of cell death, rather than cell proliferation *per se* (Kerr, Wylie and Currie, 1972; Raff, 1992; Williams, 1991; Hengartner, 1992; Carson, 1993; Evan, 1993; Millson and Malone, 1994).

The early experience of the Simontons suggests that while, on the face of it, prescribed imagery may have validity and reliability this might be quite misleading. Accordingly, the 'formulae' of guided imagery should be tested on varied populations and on a sufficiently large scale. Then modified and refined, in order to ascertain that they are both appropriate and effective for the purpose to which they are applied. However, such procedures are not generally adopted, and unlimited, untested formulae are prescribed in countless books, audio-cassettes and video-tapes, which can be purchased in the high street. In the absence of any kind of testing, the claims made for these 'preparations' are highly questionable. Furthermore, not only are they unregulated, but many of them also lack standardization.

The observations that follow are based on the author's experience of working with a series of imaginative exercises (Graham, 1992, 1995). These have been developed and standardized in a series of trials, over a number of years, involving many hundreds of people, ranging in age from 18 to 88 years.

INSTRUCTIONS ABOUT USE

Irrespective of whether a drug is prescribed or purchased over the counter, there is a legal requirement that clear and careful instructions for its use are provided. These guidelines specify when and how the drug is to be used and any contraindications. As such they reflect understanding of the way in which the drug works and what its likely effects will be.

Certain reassurances are usually included in the instructions provided with both prescribed and over-the-counter medications. These often include a brief explanation of how the medication is thought to work, and some supportive evidence, even if it is only in the form of personal testimonials. This information is important, not only in the activation of positive expectation or placebo effects, but also to relieve a person's anxieties about using the medication.

Doctors and other health professionals are generally expected to provide both information and reassurance concerning the use of the treatments they prescribe and carry out, although this is by no means standard practice. Studies (Volicer and Bohannon, 1975; Van Der Ploeg, 1988) have shown that patients perceive insufficient communication and information about medical procedures as highly stressful, with only pain being rated more so. Good health-care professionals therefore provide patients with information about the treatment prescribed, and allow sufficient time to discuss any anxieties they may have about it. All too frequently such reassurance is not given to people who are about to embark on a course of imagery exercises by authors or therapists. Nevertheless it is of considerable importance.

Guided imagery should involve guiding an individual to create a new experience for him or her, and assisting him or her in uncovering the personal meaning and significance of that experience and its relevance to their current life. In many instances, however, the guidelines provided extend only to presenting the formulae (the basic story lines for fantasy) with little or no indication as to how or when these should be used. There may be no guidance to assist the individuals to understand or cope with their responses or possible side-effects to them, or how to derive any insights from them, as a basis for personal transformation and growth. Many people who might benefit from imagery are anxious about engaging in it, because it is new to them, they have no basis for believing in its beneficial effects, and they may have misconceptions about it. A brief explanation of what imagery is and of its many applications is normally sufficient to relieve these initial anxieties. Detailed explanation of the actual process involved is usually unnecessary at the outset, as people are initially more interested in whether or not, rather than how, it works. However, as many people are both fascinated and relieved to learn that there is a rational and 'scientific' basis for what appears to be an irrational process, some indication of the possible mechanisms thought to be involved in imagery is valuable.

The nature of imagery exercises may require clarification. For some people the word exercise has connotations of physical activity, especially when it is applied in a health-related context. For others, who associate it with mental activity, it may also sound dauntingly like hard work. Explaining the point of a particular exercise is also helpful. This can be quite short and simple and open-ended, just sufficient to reassure the person that it has a purpose, without creating specific expectations. An exercise may be presented, quite simply, as directed towards greater understanding of personal needs, exploring personal potentials or whatever is the case.

It may or may not be appropriate to provide a rationale for the particular objective of an exercise. A person may not readily understand the relevance of personal needs or potentials to health or illness, for instance, and some explanation of this may be helpful. The level of explanation needs to be tailored to the sophistication of the target audience, and the degree of interest shown in details of this kind. Thus, while it might be appropriate to present health-care professionals or students with specific research findings this might be confusing for lay people.

Writers who do not include this information in their guided imagery packages should indicate sources where it can be found. Similarly, it is advisable for those working with individuals or groups in a therapeutic or educational context to be able to provide specific information or explanations if requested, or have details of sources to hand (which, of course, behoves those guiding imagery to have the requisite knowledge).

It may be more appropriate to provide this information after a particular exercise. Where this is the case it should be made quite clear to the individual concerned that this information will be provided, but that to do so beforehand might prejudice outcomes. This is usually only necessary where prior information or knowledge is likely to influence responses.

In effect, this is exactly what occurs in drug trials. In the interests of new knowledge, subjects are given little or no prior information as to the nature of a drug, other than the functions targeted. However, as in these trials, a person's right to be excluded from any unexplained procedure must be respected. Indeed it should always be made clear to subjects that participation in exercises is a matter of personal choice and that they can discontinue them whenever they wish to.

Experienced guides will be familiar with many of the issues that may be a source of anxiety for individuals about to embark on imagery exercises. They will allow ample discussion of them in books on guided imagery and in the therapeutic context.

ANTICIPATING ANXIETIES

Combining treatments

People may be anxious about the desirability or otherwise of combining imagery techniques with other forms of treatment. However, as has been noted, they are essentially used as a form of adjuvant therapy, either in support of medical treatment, psychotherapy or counselling. They are used in addition to other forms of stress management, decision making, problem solving, or creative strategies. Nevertheless, it is important to emphasize that imagery is not a substitute for conventional medical treatment or other rational strategies or *vice versa*. They are complementary but different approaches to problem solving and coping.

Being unimaginative

Many people consider themselves to be unimaginative, and are anxious that imaginative methods will be difficult or even impossible for them. As a result, some will not attempt imagery, while others who do so anticipate negative outcomes and failure. It would seem that in many cases people associate being imaginative with intellectual activities, having been told by their teachers in childhood that they lack imagination in their schoolwork.

People generally do not identify their ability to see things 'in the mind's eye' with imagination, regarding the former as quite natural and commonplace, and the latter as a more specialized talent, possessed by relatively few. Nor do they readily appreciate to what extent the planning, coordination and execution of their everyday lives depends on the ability to create mental images. Indeed, the planning and execution of mundane activities would be almost impossible without this ability. When it is pointed out that people choose and coordinate what they wear; how they decorate and furnish their homes; landscape their gardens; select their holiday destination from those advertised in a brochure, and much else, largely on the basis of their ability to create, mix and match images in their minds, anxieties about being unimaginative are usually greatly relieved.

Nevertheless, some people remain convinced that they are less imaginative than others, especially when they hear others relate their imagery in group situations. It is therefore important to emphasize that some people are more 'visile' than others, as Galton first noted in 1883. Those whose visual imagery is not strong and who experience difficulty in generating or holding detailed images generally overcome these difficulties with practice. Imagery is not necessarily visual – auditory, tactile, olfactory, gustatory and kinaesthetic images are equally valid and important. Indeed, imagery exercises should guide individuals to become fully aware not only of sights, but also sounds, smells and other sensations. It should also be emphasized that most people require practice before producing vivid imagery, and that initially images are often vague and weak. Furthermore, those whose imagery remains weak despite practice should not be obliged to employ visual imagery, but encouraged to use the imagerial mode with which they feel most comfortable and to experience it as fully as possible.

Many people have difficulty in recognizing what constitutes imagery, or acknowledging their imagery as a product of the imagination. Some believe that unless their images are wholly invented they are not truly imaginary. Others show considerable confusion between objective and subjective realities. They may insist that, because an object or scene they visualize has a real-life counterpart, their imagery is objective and 'real' rather than a subjective mental representation of these features of the outer world. Others fail to recognize that much of what they take to be real in the world is imaginary. They tend to regard reality as an immutable, objective domain outside of themselves, in some way fixed and beyond their control. They fail to recognize the extent to which they create that reality through their beliefs, assumptions, expectations and imaginings, and thus the degree of choice they have in determining their lives. Moreover, because the events and circumstances of their lives appear fixed, and their responses to them unavoidable, stress is perceived as an inevitability rather than a choice. For such people, the idea implicit in guided imagery that one can create a different reality by cultivating a different outlook or attitude, or by seeing things in a different light, and may as a result be able to solve problems and reduce or eliminate stress, is often very difficult to grasp.

Similarly, those who fail to recognize that their imagery is not 'real' may not readily appreciate that other 'realities' of their existence, such as fears, anxieties, expectations and assumptions, self and body images and identity, may also be wholly or in part imaginary, and a source of unnecessary and avoidable difficulties and stress. Indeed, for many people 'reality', comprising as it does, fantasised ideas about the self, others and the world, imaginary threats and fears, is largely fantasy. Most of their problems result from the fact that they are 'hooked' on this fantasy and cannot distinguish it from reality. Aggression, for example, often arises as a response to an imagined insult, and fear may arise through anticipated rather than actual danger.

Ernst and Goodison (1981) therefore counter the claim that the energy expended in fantasy would be better utilized in coming to terms with reality. They point out that by using imagery, individuals are able to confront and accept the reality of who and what they are, rather than their fantasy ideals. Exposing and exploring rather than ignoring fantasy prevents people being bound up in fantasies. Guided imagery or fantasy can therefore be used to contact qualities within the self, to express personal power and potentials, and to enable action in the real world. Accordingly, they suggest, individuals can move from a situation where their dreams frighten them, their fantasies dominate their waking life, and anxieties cut them off from the world, to a situation where they have more of their personal power available to live their lives creatively in the present.

Performance anxiety

Many people are concerned whether they will be able to 'do' the exercises correctly. Anxiety that they might not, often translates into muscular tension and may be sufficient to inhibit relaxation and the production of imagery. This response may reflect a general anxiety about performance, achievement, success, failure or evaluation and the way these generate tensions in people's lives and limit their experience. It can promote valuable insights if highlighted by a guide.

Everyone embarking on imagery should be advised that imagery is not a matter of 'doing' anything so much as of 'being' open and receptive to aspects of the self which emerge when the pressure to 'do' is relaxed. Consequently trying to do imagery is counterproductive, and needs to be abandoned in favour of 'allowing' imagery to emerge spontaneously, and allowing sufficient time for this to occur.

Another common concern expressed by those who produce imagery is that they might be doing so incorrectly because they imagine themselves in scenes in a detached manner, as though looking down on themselves. This in no way reduces the potency or validity of the imagery, and is quite usual initially. Indeed many people use imagery very effectively without ever becoming fully immersed in it.

Generally, people experience very little difficulty in generating imagery, and find it pleasurable, although they may also find it puzzling at times. Some, finding their imagination 'playing odd tricks', that is, producing unexpected imagery or that which they regard as unacceptable to themselves or others, may attempt to censor or direct it more conventionally. This kind of censorship is not only very common but also potentially very significant, providing as it does, clues to the moral and other imperatives that shape a person's life and his or her responses to it. Effective guides will draw attention to its importance.

It is particularly important to instruct those working with imagery to avoid the tendency consciously to direct or to censor it. To do so is to impose the strictures of the conscious rational mind rather than to allow unconscious contents to emerge and defeats the whole point of the exercise. People should therefore be encouraged to be aware of the first image that comes spontaneously to mind, whether it is a picture, a sound, word, scent or other sensation. They should allow sufficient time for it to be clarified and amplified, attempting neither to hold on to it and thus resist the formation of other images, nor seizing other images as they emerge and failing to allow any of them to develop fully. The aim of imaginative approaches is to give a free rein to the imagination, therefore deviation from the prescribed images, which are merely a spur to the imagination, is to be encouraged.

Mind wandering

Allowing the imagination to 'run free' is achieved by reducing the volume of conscious thoughts, such as everyday anxieties, concerns and preoccupations which dominate ordinary thinking, much as a jockey controls a racehorse. The prospect of giving rein to the imagination creates real anxiety in many people, and the jockey (their conscious mind) attempts to gain greater control, tightening his grip on the reins, and turning the horse around and about itself so that it cannot make any progress forward, and he is carried round in circles. The mind wanders around in much the same way for many people when they begin imagery exercises, turning again and again to certain issues, and frustrating progress in generating imagery.

This problem can be aggravated by certain medical conditions and pain, which may be overriding concerns for people. Where this problem occurs, and it does so commonly, progressive physical relaxation is often recommended. However, unless the person can relax or let go of the mental tensions generating the problem this proves self-defeating. One of the author's clients reported that he had tried every conceivable method of relaxation and could achieve physical relaxation to the extent of losing all awareness of his body, at which point he invariably became aware of the contents of his mind (financial worries) and immediately became tense again.

Recognition of precisely this kind of difficulty led Perls to encourage his clients to 'lose their minds' in the ordinary sense. It was for much the same purpose (that of letting go of or suspending conscious thought) that Jung advo-cated the practice of active imagination. However, the fear of losing their mind, in any sense may be a major source of anxiety for many people.

Losing control

Fear of losing control is very common, and to some people this is implied in the notion of suppressing consciousness in any way, however transiently. Others worry that by doing so they may become unconscious. Both ideas are fostered by misconceptions about hypnosis, which is commonly portrayed as a trance-like state in which the person loses awareness and becomes subject to control by the hypnotists. This highly misleading view is perpetuated by popular writers, the media, stage performers and some professional hypnotists. Yet during hypnosis awareness is not lost. If anything, awareness is enhanced, and this is equally true of imagery. Moreover, self-control increases. Indeed, letting go of the constraints normally imposed on the body by rational conscious processes may enable people not only to become aware of, but also to influence directly, physiological processes ordinarily beyond conscious control. This is, in effect, how hypnosis and other imagery methods achieve their effects.

Becoming irrational

For some people becoming 'lost' in fantasy is a genuine anxiety. They fear that they might lose themselves by looking inwards. Within Western culture introver-sion is largely synonymous with shyness and frequently carries the connotation of weakness. It is therefore widely regarded as an undesirable trait which produces withdrawn and other-worldly people who gradually lose touch with reality. Not uncommonly it is associated with madness, especially schizophrenia.

This general view is reflected in Western medicine. Indeed, the confusion in both lay and medical circles between the characteristics common to mysticism and mental disorder, prompted the US Group for the Advancement of Psychiatry to attempt a clarification which was reported in *The Practitioner* in 1977. This indicated that any resemblance between the mystic and the schizo-phrenic is merely superficial. The retreat of the former into the inner world being deliberate rather than obligatory, partial rather than complete, and there-fore controlled rather than uncontrolled. However, the report failed to make any absolute distinction between mysticism and mental disturbance, and, if anything, further confused the issue by concluding that 'from one point of view all mystical experiences may be regarded as symptoms of mental disturbance, and from another, they may be regarded as attempts at adaption'. Hamachek makes a more useful distinction, observing that the capacity to remove oneself temporarily from unpleasant realities of the physical world into a more affable world of fantasy has considerable therapeutic value, and is problematic only when a person uses it as a permanent escape from reality. As he indicates, it is one thing to build a castle in the sky and quite another to try to live in it (Hamachek, 1971, p. 20).

Being immature

A common fear, shared by both sexes, is of being thought childish or silly. This fear relates not merely to the content of a person's imagery but to the process of imagination itself. Some people are reluctant to engage in it or admit to doing so, while others adopt cynical, sceptical or dismissive attitudes towards it. The limiting effect this may have on personal experience is considerable. It was highlighted for the author during a professional training course when a woman, who was clearly reluctant to engage in an exercise, admitted being unhappy about being asked to 'play about' with a certain idea. She considered that this trivialized the issue, and her, because her time was being wasted by it. Asked to elaborate on her concept of play, she indicated that it is something quite incompatible with work, and not to be treated seriously. It was pointed out to her that play is the means by which young humans and animals learn about their environment and themselves, and as such is crucial to cognitive development. Moreover, play deprivation impairs intellectual development and functioning, so rather than being in any sense wasteful, it is highly productive and creative. Thus reassured that the enterprise she was being asked to engage in was not belittling, she consented to continue with it.

Given what is now known about the physiology of laughter and its beneficial effects on health, and the undesirable health consequences of psychological rigidity, this suppression of fun and playfulness is somewhat alarming. The concern not to be childish is suggestive of a rather tenuous self-identity and maturity. Hence this woman's concerns about engaging in play potentially reveal a good deal about her state of health.

Using guided imagery with children

Concern about the childishness or silliness of imagery exercises sometimes prompts the question of their applicability to children. Psychological research has shown that children who are imaginative tend to score more highly in tests of intellectual ability and are better able to cope than children who are unimaginative. Encouraging imagination, creativity and self-expression also improves the ability to cope and learn (Oaklander, 1978). It is for this reason that play, and all kinds of imaginary activities, including visualization and guided fantasy, are increasingly being used by teachers at all educational levels. Imagery is also being used increasingly in therapy, not only with those who have learning difficulties but also with those who are emotionally disturbed.

In advocating the therapeutic uses of imagery in working with children, Oaklander explains that the fantasy process of a child is usually the same as his or her life process. Therefore, 'We can look into the inner realms of the child's being through fantasy. We can bring out what is kept hidden or avoided and we can also find out what's going on in the child's life, from her perspective'. Ways of doing so include not only guided imagery but also forms of story-telling, writing, painting, drawing, modelling, poetry and puppetry. Oaklander observes that simply by drawing a picture of a fantasy and writing a summary statement of it, children may indicate very succinctly where they are in their lives, and their feelings about it. This approach is used to access children's feelings and to enable them to become aware of themselves and their existence in the world. It is considered particularly appropriate in dealing with stress, trauma, phobias and issues that children have difficulty expressing.

Guided imagery, in particular, may be very useful in developing what McKellar (1989) terms 'empathy bridges', not only between teacher or therapist and child, but also between parent(s) and child. Roet (cited Jackson, 1993) advocates the use of imagery as a means whereby parents can gain insight into the normally hidden realms of their children's experience (their fears, anxieties, needs, wishes and preoccupations) and thus monitor emotional and psychological development more sensitively. Like Oaklander, he believes that for children fantasy is reality, and that for them 'the inner world of pictures', which as adults they often have to rediscover, 'is already there' rather than created by technique. He suggests that on a superficial or 'conscious' level children have symptoms, feelings or attitudes that are mirrored in the internal world of pictures, and that changes in the latter will bring about parallel changes at the conscious level. He also believes that parents and teachers can easily learn the basic skills of listening to and validating children's fantasies, and, by relating to them on their own level, help them through various crises.

Losing the soul

Some people fear that by looking inwards into the hidden or 'occult' aspects of themselves, or others, they will encounter evil and terrible features, and lose their souls rather than their minds. Such fears are often encouraged by ministers of religion and others who view this ordinarily hidden domain as the realm of the devil. Jung referred to these features as the 'shadow', describing this as everything that a person refuses to acknowledge about him or herself, and which a person typically defends or protects against in various ways, most usually by keeping it hidden. It is because their hidden, darker or 'shadowy' features are often considered crazy, evil or sinful that people may wish not simply to hide, but to rid themselves of them. However, as Jung (1954, Vol. 9 Part 2, p. 266) has indicated:

> If it has been believed hitherto that the human shadow was the source of all evil, it can now be ascertained on closer investigation that the uncon-scious man, that is, his shadow, does not consist only of morally repre-hensible tendencies, but also displays a number of good qualities, such as

normal instincts, appropriate reactions, realistic insights, creative impulses.

For Jung it is less a matter or ridding oneself of the shadow than of learning to live with it. Accordingly, Jung conceived of psychotherapy as concerned with helping a person to explore the hinterland of his mind, and to grow by confronting and making contact with the dissociated aspects of the self:

> The aim is to observe the sporadic emergence, whether in the form of images or feelings, of those dim representations which detach themselves in the darkness from the invisible realm of the unconscious and move as shadows before the inturned gaze. In this way things repressed and forgotten come back again. This is a gain in itself, though often a painful one (Jung, 1954, Vol. 16, p. 59).

Jung insisted that man's confrontation with his shadow must be brought into consciousness (brought into the light as it were) and recognized, before it can be integrated with the conscious self. This process is a necessary step in the movement towards completion, wholeness or health. His view can perhaps be summed up in the modern idiom: 'no pain, no gain'. Certainly, as is the case with many medicines and other forms of treatment, the experience of imagery may be emotionally painful, unpalatable or unpleasant and may be strongly resisted. However, as Jung observed, it is towards oneself that one has the strongest resistances. It is invariably the case that when these are examined they reveal negative beliefs about the self. The Simontons (Simonton and Simonton, 1975) emphasize the importance of the person's belief systems in achieving successful outcomes. They insist that negative beliefs and expectancies can only be changed if they are brought to the surface.

ANTICIPATING RESISTANCE

In addition to providing adequate information and assurance to those about to embark on imagery, an effective guide should be able to identify resistance and help people to overcome it. The Simontons indicate that some people are unwilling or unable to engage in imagery because they feel that to imagine their cancer shrinking when they have been told that it is actually growing constitutes lying. This concern is general to all the applications of guided imagery rather than just its therapeutic uses. It is important for the guide to emphasize that mental imagery is 'not a method of self-deception; it is a means of self-direction' (Simonton, Matthews-Simonton and Creighton, 1978, p. 139); and that what is being imagined is the desired outcome rather than what is happening at the time.

However, as the Simontons indicate, a preoccupation with physical illness may conceal a strong fear of the disease and doubt about the body's ability to overcome it. Similarly preoccupation with aches and pains, minor irritations, noises, draughts and the like are typical ways in which people avoid engaging in imagery. Such avoidance invariably conceals a person's resistance to looking into him- or herself. Simply identifying these tendencies as possible avoidance strategies may help a person to become aware of this resistance, and is therefore potentially important.

Some people readily acknowledge that they do not want to look too closely at the hidden or unknown aspects of themselves, either out of fear of what they will find, or because of the implications it might have for their lives. It is therefore also important for a guide to recognize that many people will hold on to their problems, including potentially life-threatening illnesses, rather than take responsibility for change. Guides should encourage people to confront the consequences of change that they fear.

Siegel (1986), a noted surgeon and Assistant Clinical Professor of Surgery at Yale Medical School, estimates that when given a choice between surgery for serious illness and a change in lifestyle, 80% will opt for the former, because it demands no action on their part, transfers responsibility elsewhere, and maintains the status quo. Coronary patients are also reluctant to examine their basic problems (Friedman and Rosenman, 1974). Cancer patients typically resist doing so even more strongly, usually because of negative views and beliefs about themselves (Simonton, 1983).

Others will deny being reluctant to look at themselves or their problems. Indeed they may not be conscious of this avoidance tendency. However, it is frequently revealed in their reactions to working with imagery. Some people make the excuse that they 'got nowhere' with the exercises because they 'drifted off' or 'fell asleep'. Sleep, rather like illness, is all too often an excuse for inactivity and a way of excusing responsibility for tasks the person does not wish to perform. It is a classic way of avoiding personal potentials or other features of the self, and the responsibilities and fears that attach to them. Domestic and zoo animals frequently curl up and sleep when stressed in some way, presumably on the principle that if they lie quietly or play 'doggo' the threat will go away. Humans react similarly when their cages are rattled. As John le Carré has observed, 'By changing nothing we hang on to what we understand, even if it is the bars of our own gaol' (*The Russia House*, p. 122).

Being 'rattled' occasionally can be liberating, and closer examination of images that evoke this reaction is to be encouraged. Nevertheless, it has to be recognized that the very idea of imagework challenges or compromises the belief systems of some people, and may compromise their view of themselves in significant ways.

Some people believe that it is wrong for them to engage in a pleasurable indulgence or interesting diversion such as imagery, when there are other things they should be doing. This kind of self-denial is potentially very significant because the 'shoulds' and 'should nots' of people's lives often generate stress and illness. All too frequently one encounters women who cannot allow themselves to relax because they should be looking after others, and men who believe that they must work around the clock to support others, and must not take time off for themselves. Even if they give themselves permission to take some time for themselves and relax, these self-imposed imperatives often prevent them doing so effectively. Therefore people need to be guided to identify and examine the rules of conduct they impose on themselves and the anxieties and problems generated thereby.

A common observation among those who use guided imagery in therapy, especially in the treatment of physical illness, is that women are more prone to discontinue exercises than men. This is because to take time 'off' for what they regard as a self-indulgent activity compromises their view of themselves as proper wives, mothers and so on. Men are therefore more likely to use imagery more effectively (Manning, 1988). However, fewer men are attracted to and use the approach, presumably because it compromises their view of themselves as mature, rational people.

Some people state quite simply that they cannot imagine whatever it is they are asked to. Rather than merely accepting that this is the case, it is important for them to examine what is stopping them doing so. Examination often reveals that the particular image compromises a person's view of him or herself, or other beliefs they hold. Men, for example, may declare a particular image unmanly, which is itself significant as it reflects stereotypical assumptions about what is or is not appropriate, and the kinds of restrictions they impose even on their most private experience. These limiting factors are often at the root of many of their problems and difficulties. Inability to produce images because of their possible feminine connotations, for example, suggests a very frail masculine identity. Accordingly close examination of images that people find difficulty accepting and wish to change, and the reasons behind this, is desirable.

Similarly it is appropriate to alert people who ordinarily have little or no difficulty in generating imagery to the possible significance of finding themselves unable to 'do' a certain exercise, and the explanations or excuses they offer if and when this occurs. They might, for example, respond to an exercise which asks them to imagine the sea by saying that they don't like, or are frightened by water, and for this reason were unable to 'get into' an exercise it which it features. Irrespective of any symbolic significance that water might have for them, such a response serves to highlight the way in which conscious preconceived views restrict experience even at the fantasy level, and the extent to which certain expectations and beliefs impose limits on their experience by preventing them exploring different responses or creating new experiences for themselves.

Some people may resist imagery because they do not want to become better. As with other forms of avoidance or resistance the underlying issues need to be brought to the surface. Pointing out to people that they might be avoiding looking at aspects of themselves and their lives is, however, different from trying to force them to look at these things. They should be encouraged to do so at a time and pace that is appropriate for them. This may involve them deferring doing so. It is by no means uncommon for people to 'give up' imagery, whether self-help courses or otherwise, only to return to it at a later time when they feel more prepared for the self-scrutiny it demands.

Some people believe that they will not be able to 'do' the exercises correctly on their own. Others think they cannot achieve results by themselves and that they need people to help them. Many of these people therefore prefer to attend therapy, courses of exercises or workshops, rather than to continue on a self-help basis. These reasons may be a significant factor in the greater effectiveness of therapist-led relaxation and imagery compared with self-help audio-cassettes and the like. Some audiotapes chosen as an aid to relaxation give the misleading impression that relaxation is easily and quickly achieved. Those who, on using them, find that this is not the case can easily become discouraged, conclude that they cannot relax, and give up trying altogether. Similarly, people who find it difficult to visualize what they are instructed to, may conclude that they are incapable of imagery. Such 'aids' are clearly counterproductive. Nevertheless, audiotapes are valuable in helping people to remember an exercise, especially when these are long and/or complex, and they overcome the distractions which result from trying to follow an exercise while reading it. For this reason recording of exercises is advisable for those using imaginative exercises on a self-help basis. Ideally, exercises should be developed and written with this in mind.

PREPARATION FOR GUIDED IMAGERY

In some cases anxiety and resistance can be remedied by relaxation. Achterberg (1985) claims that deep relaxation is necessary to prevent motor responses, thoughts and external stimuli competing with the production of imagery. She regards any kind of relaxation as suitable, providing that it is not too wordy, not longer than 20 minutes duration, and that the setting is suitable, inasmuch as it does not generate or increase anxiety. She therefore considers hospitals as generally unsuitable settings for imagery-based methods.

Arguably, however, while these conditions are desirable they are not essential. Ordinarily, deep relaxation is not a necessary prerequisite of imagery, although it might be in instances where a person is hypertense. For most people absorption in imagery is sufficient to promote relaxation, which is an important consideration in cases where pain prevents progressive physical relaxation.

Moreover, Snyder (1984) draws attention to certain possible contraindications to the use of progressive relaxation. He suggests that it may cause greater withdrawal in depressed persons; that the tropotrophic state created by relaxation may intensify the toxic effects of certain medications and may result in hypotensive or hypoglycaemic reactions; and that cardiac patients should be advised against tensing muscles tightly. In addition, people with a history of psychiatric disorder characterized by problems of self-control, may become intensely anxious as a result of relaxation, as might those with suicidal tendencies.

Furthermore, the wordiness of relaxation methods would appear to be largely irrelevant given that as relaxation progresses most people spontaneously 'turn off' or 'screen out' these external stimuli. For this reason the setting in which imagery exercises are undertaken is also largely irrelevant. It is perhaps worth noting that the author has successfully guided imagery in: a busy hospital ward; an unsound-proofed glass building adjacent to a town fire station during a period when the fire brigade was noisily summoned several times; in various buildings where fire or burglar alarms or ambulance sirens have sounded; in a room over a dance studio where an enthusiastic aerobics group was working out to rock and pop music and literally raising the roof; in at least two rooms where there has been a sudden and complete failure of power and heating; and during several thunderstorms and gales.

Indeed, people generally seem more troubled by the presence of strangers or too many friends and acquaintances than the setting *per se* when initially engaging in imagery. Comfort, both physical and psychological, is more important than context. It is therefore appropriate to recommend that people intending to engage in imagery exercises find somewhere they can feel safe, comfortable and able to relax, either alone, or in the company of selected others.

Paradoxically, however, too much comfort is undesirable as it tends to induce sleep. For this reason it is advisable to recommend that people sit rather than lie down when engaging in imagery. Ideally, the body will be well supported, with both feet set apart and firmly on the ground, arms resting along the arms of a chair or the thighs, and no parts of the body twisted or crossed. Restrictive clothing should be loosened and shoes and spectacles removed.

It might be assumed that it is necessary to close the eyes before engaging in imagery, while this may facilitate the process, it is not an absolute requirement. It is advisable for people wearing contact lenses not to close their eyes, as this will lead to discomfort. Also, some people, because of congenital defect, surgery or injury, cannot close their eyes. In such cases focusing the eyes on a fixed point throughout the imagery exercise will effectively reduce competing visual stimulation.

FREQUENCY OF USE

Ideally the period(s) of time allocated to these methods will be determined on the basis of what appears most beneficial to the individual, the purpose for which they are being used, and the ease with which any particular regime can be built into daily routine. Guidance on this issue is not always provided, and many people are concerned as to how long they should spend on any exercise; how frequently exercises should be undertaken; and whether exercises should be repeated.

The Simontons initially recommended three daily periods of approximately 20 minutes each, and this regime is still advocated for those who are using imagery in the treatment of physical illness. Where it is employed for relaxation, self-awareness, spiritual development or problem solving other times may be appropriate. Normally, 20–30 minutes each day is sufficient for an imagery exercise, preferably not just before retiring for the night, as the person is likely to fall asleep. However, the most appropriate time is that which suits the individual. Many people find it difficult to find a time which suits them and adhere to it every day, and for this reason often prefer to join a weekly class or therapy group. However, this is unlikely to confer many benefits if it is the sole period devoted to imagery in a week; a point which requires emphasis, along with the importance of regular homework.

KEEPING RECORDS

Repetition of exercises is desirable because the insights they afford will alter as the person's life situation changes. Often people quite wrongly assume that an exercise will produce the same images and the same insights however many times it is repeated. This is rarely the case (and where it is, the possibility that this represents resistance to the emergence of new insights and change is suggested). When similar imagery is evoked on successive trials novel and/or additional insights usually emerge also. For this reason, and because imagery, whether that of dreams or deliberate fantasy, however intense or significant, is only fleeting and quickly forgotten, it is desirable that individuals make some record of their responses to any particular exercise. It is also important that the verbal representational mode is brought to bear on visually represented issues, and that verbal and non-verbal processes are integrated. The record may be in the form of an audio-recording or written log book. The former has the advantages of greater immediacy and speed, and affords considerable detail, but it may not always be convenient. Moreover, it restricts the record to verbal content, whereas the point of imagework is to integrate verbal and non-verbal modes of consciousness and enhance communication between them. Von Franz (1975) suggests that written dialogue often produces the best results.

However, a verbal and visual record of experiences, in both words and pictures, which incorporates sketches and paintings, is more appropriate to what might be regarded traditionally as a 'vision quest'. Macbeth (1991) recommends what she terms an 'image dictionary' (perhaps more appropriately a pictionary) as a useful appendix to this record. She suggests that interpretations of specific images are recorded separately so that each person begins to build up his or her own symbolic vocabulary. She also makes the important observation that these images do not need to make 'sense'; there may not be conscious, verbal, connections between the images and the subjects they represent. It is sufficient simply to know who or what is represented by a particular symbol, so that when it is encountered subsequently, in dreams or elsewhere, it is recognized as having some bearing on feelings about, and relations with that particular subject.

Certain features of imagery tend to recur in different contexts and detail in the course of a series of exercises so that what initially may appear obscure, meaningless or trivial becomes progressively more clear, intelligible, relevant and significant. The record should therefore include details of incidental and coincidental material. These include experiences and insights which occur as a result of the exercises rather than during them, such as when a feature or theme arising in an exercise recurs or is amplified in a subsequent dream, reverie or actual life experience. 'Coincidences' such as these are invariably highly significant but are often overlooked or dismissed. Frequently people subsequently discover in a book, magazine or newspaper an exact, or almost exact, representation of their images. Inclusion of illustrative material such as this in the record is desirable because it not only jogs the memory but also helps to clarify thoughts about imagery and to facilitate interpretation of them.

Images may produce 'side-effects' inasmuch as they tend to stimulate a good deal of thought long after the exercises are over and stimulate other unconscious processes such as dreaming. It is therefore not unusual to encounter the same motifs or symbols in subsequent dreams, daydreams or fantasies. Thus a dream may yield further understanding of a previously unfathomed image; just as an imagery exercise may clarify the content of a dream. Indeed it would appear that once the 'bridge' between the conscious and unconscious aspects of the self has been opened, the unconscious will take every opportunity to use it. Dreaming typically becomes more frequent and more vivid (those who have not previously dreamed in colour may find that they begin to do so) and impresses itself more powerfully on the individual. The entire imaginal system seems to develop and become elaborated.

The meaning of certain images may be discerned as a result of other activities, in sudden flashbacks of images, or flashes of insight, which in some cases may be dramatic. Whereas this latter 'Eureka' effect usually brings about a sudden transformation of consciousness, understanding or awareness, images may recur without any increased insight or understanding. These should not be dismissed or ignored, but carefully noted. Usually resolution will occur quite spontaneously, but as with medical symptoms which persist despite treatment, it is advisable to seek assistance if troubling images persist for an appreciable time.

A record helps to identify certain patterns in a person's life and experience by highlighting significant issues or 'themes', and encourages greater self-awareness. Importantly, it also helps cultivate a disciplined approach to self-examination. A record of this kind is particularly important if images are being deliberately rehearsed, as in therapeutic approaches, such as those advocated by the Simontons, or to improve performance, as in the case of sport, other skilled activity, or rehabilitation, where certain outcomes are desired. In such cases, it is advisable to establish that the images employed are appropriate to the task in hand.

Macbeth (1991) likens this record to the grimoire or working notebook in which a sorcerer or magician enters details of journeys into inner worlds. She observes that 'this journal does not need to be a literary masterpiece or work of art. In fact, it will probably be more honest if it is neither of those things' (Macbeth, 1991, p. 11). Keeping such a record over a course of exercises is valuable because the effects of imagery tend to be progressive and cumulative. It is essentially an aide-memoire, enabling a person to refer back to earlier images, and to keep track of both process and progress. However, as Macbeth indicates, its most important use is in the present moment; helping the person to understand what is happening now.

For this, and other reasons, it is desirable to record imagery verbally in the first person, present tense. The personalization of imagery, which results from its description in this way, not only locates the experience in the immediate present but also helps to reverse any tendency towards projection, whereby responsibility for personal creations or products (whether imaginings, thoughts, feelings, pains, actions or illnesses) is attributed to external causes. This projection of personal features onto the outside world and others gives rise to the idea that these external forces are responsible for, or cause them. Typically people use phrases such as 'it makes me angry', or 'sick', rather than 'I make myself angry' or 'sick' in response to who or whatever it might be. Even more impersonal is the use of the word 'one'. In both cases a verbal ploy distances people from themselves as a source of their feelings and responsibility for them, implying that their source is external and beyond personal control. The personalization of images and feelings brought about by the use of the first person, present tense works in reverse. It helps to promote acknowledgement of personal responsibility and locus of control; that is, the sense of being effective in the world rather than a passive victim of circumstance, and awareness of one's contribution to problems and illnesses.

This verbal shift also helps to highlight the possible significance of imagery. People will frequently deny that there is any, arguing that the image corresponds to some feature of the 'real' world. However, while it may correspond with a feature of the external world it is nevertheless a product of their imagination and its potential significance lies in why, of all the features of the world they could have brought to mind or invented, they chose to represent this one. The person needs to be encouraged to recognize it as a specific personal production or creation for which they are responsible, and which, for this very reason is almost certainly meaningful when scrutinized more closely.

Those who cannot readily see the personal relevance of an image when viewed objectively may feel quite differently when they personalize it or 'try it on'. Thus translated, for example, 'I imagine a cool, unmoving pool with murky depths' becomes 'I am a cool, unmoving pool with murky depths', which at the very least gives food for thought.

The majority of people are only too clearly aware that their images are significant, although they may not be able to discern what their meaning is. They tend to look outside themselves for answers and solutions rather than within. This reflects not only the tendency to project responsibility outside themselves, but also the extrovert or outward looking tendency of Western culture, which encourages respect for authorities and experts, especially in the health field. However, the major challenge of self-help, especially as regards health, is for individuals to assume the responsibility to become, and to acknowledge themselves as the ultimate authority on themselves.

Nevertheless, as the Simontons realized, and indicated in their pioneering work in the medical uses of imagery, frequently the meanings of a person's images, whether spontaneous or responses to prescribed stimuli, are not readily discerned by the individual, and they need help in translating what is essentially a unique symbolic vocabulary. Without this assistance much of the purpose of imagery is lost, and people are frequently left puzzled, confused, alarmed, and in some instances, distressed by images and accompanying powerful feelings they are unable to understand. Furthermore, where 'untranslated' images are rehearsed without comprehension of their full meaning, the resulting outcome may be far from what is intended or desired, especially if the images are inappropriate for the task in hand. A case in point would be the repetition of imagery which is self-defeating or futile. For example, that of a woman who repeatedly imagined her body's healing forces energetically spraying foam over a virulent weed to no effect whatever, until she realized that the foam was not a powerful herbicide as she had at first thought, but merely soap. Similarly, 'smuggled assumptions' (delimiting and negative thoughts) (Gellatly, 1986) are likely to undermine the likelihood of positive outcomes and effects from imagery. For example, in the case of the man whose healing 'force', mobilized in an attempt to prevent the spread of a rapidly advancing cancer, comprised two men blocking off a tunnel on an underground railway track with the benefit of only a portable cement-mixer, a bucket and two spades. Use of inappropriate imagery in this way may lead to its dismissal by some people as pointless, valueless and ineffective; and by others as potentially damaging and harmful. Neither view is likely to persuade health-care professionals of the possible therapeutic benefits of such methods.

IMAGE EXPLICATION

The novelist E.M. Forster penned the maxim 'only connect', and this is the fundamental principle of image explication. Shotter (1975, p. 42), describes it as 'the attempt to characterize as clearly and as systematically as possible the nature of a person's imagery'. The information conveyed by images is generally, although not exclusively, non-verbal, non-linear, non-sequential and non-discrete. Accordingly it requires integration rather than summation; synthesis rather than analysis. Jung, somewhat paradoxically, described his therapeutic approach as both 'analytical' and 'complex' inasmuch as it was directed towards analysis of elements of the psyche and reshaping the whole. Accordingly, Hochheimer (1969) suggested that Jung's methods should be described as 'spagyric', a term which derives from the Greek terms *span*, meaning to separate into component parts, and *ageiren*, meaning to assemble. As such they are similar to that involved in the completion of jigsaw puzzles. Working with imagery can be likened to puzzling over a vast jigsaw, and trying to establish the connections between its many features (Graham, 1995). This is achieved primarily by identifying the association or links between elements. Simple word association may be effective, but the tendency to generate lists of words should be avoided. It is preferable to 'brain-storm' by writing or drawing the image or its component features in the centre of a large piece of paper or blackboard and then generating associations (both verbal and pictorial) to each of the associations as they are produced. Each associated item can be 'mapped' on to the paper, by placing each one, as it emerges, close to the word or picture that triggered it, until no further associations can be made (or the available space is used up). In this way, thousands of items may be generated, each linked to others. The connections between items can then be made by joining them. This invariably results in a huge circular plan, not unlike a mandala, or web, which features both straight and curved lines. As such it represents a cognitive 'map' of multiple, simultaneous and multi-sensory associations very different from that which results from listing verbal or memory associations.

Drawing, painting, various kinds of artwork and colour can be incorporated into this mental map, which may be used not only in the amplification and elaboration of images but for generating ideas, planning essays and stimulating creative thinking of all kinds. Nevertheless, most people have been educated and trained to organize their thoughts linearly, in lists and flow diagrams, and usually require a good deal of guidance, encouragement and practice before they feel comfortable with this unusual procedure, and can use it effectively.

Frequently, images generate both verbal and visual puns, which should be included in the map. Puns and ambiguities are often highly significant and images often repay careful examination. An example from personal experience may illustrate this. In a visit to *The Magic Shop* (Graham, 1992) the author realized that the long white apron in which the shopkeeper was attired would not have been imagined were it not in some way significant, but despite repeated attempts was unable to fathom its meaning. Much later, after various associations had been produced, the apron was recognized as a cobbler's apron, but again the significance of this continued to be elusive until the question, 'what does a cobbler do?' provoked the answer, 'he mends soles'. Through recognizing this as a pun, it became clear that the doorkeeper was in fact involved with the repair of souls – psychotherapy – a highly significant issue for the author who was, at that time, planning a book on the subject. However, a former student suggested an alternative interpretation of the imagery; that it was merely 'cobblers'!

Images can be worked on in many other ways. One of the most striking illustrations of some of these is presented in Steven Speilberg's film *Close Encounters of the Third Kind*, where the hero attempts to clarify a vague mental impression he has formed of a landscape by drawing, modelling in clay (and mashed potato), earthworking and various other constructions. In this way he refines the image sufficiently to be able to recognize its 'real-life' counterpart when this is shown briefly on television. This is a classic example of the way in which coincidence often serves to amplify, illuminate and resolve puzzling imagery.

Imaginary scenes may be dramatized, using cartoon figures, puppets, dolls, toys, other persons, or by the individual acting out or talking through each of the 'parts' of the fantasy in turn. Role-play games can be elaborated around the themes or characters of imagery, and board games can be developed for this purpose.

Gestalt-style techniques may be used to project the various elements of the imagery into empty chairs so as to interact with them and engage them in dialogue; or to 'shuttle' between the manifest content of the imagery and the associations it evokes.

Many of these methods can be used by individuals when working alone or with others and guided by books and other media, or when guided directly by others on a one-to-one or group basis. In this way people may begin to recognize and understand elements of their personal symbolism, and the meanings of themes in which certain symbols recur. However, irrespective of how individuals work with imagery, or who works with them, they should always be alert to the possibility of any tendency towards over-prescription by their guide(s).

OVER-PRESCRIPTION

Over-prescription may occur in two ways. Over-direction of a person's imagery may occur when the guide, consciously or unconsciously, suggests certain images to a person. Alternatively, the guide may make definitive interpretations of the images generated by an individual.

Over-directive guidance

The specific purpose of guided imagery is for the individual to discover the meanings he or she has projected into essentially neutral stimuli in the form of symbols or vague storylines provided by another. It can be thought of as a process whereby a bare outline or 'storyboard' is provided as the basis of a 'movie' in the mind, which the individual then casts, enacts, produces, directs and subsequently reviews. By doing this the person confronts the ordinarily unconscious or unrecognized aspects of the self, making them conscious, so that these insights can be related directly to life.

A fine line exists between a 'storyboard' which provides a basis for projection by the individual, and one which provides too much personal projection by the guide, and is already coloured by his or her imagination. For example, when guiding a fantasy much less 'creating' one, it is all too easy to allow features that are seen in one's own mind's eye to 'contaminate' the pictures formed by another. Similarly, someone guiding an exercise may personalize what should be neutral elements of it simply by referring to them as persons rather than figures; or by attributing gender to them through the use of the pronouns he or she. Although subtle, these terms guide the imagination in very specific ways, foreclosing it and eliminating other spontaneous responses that might be generated by a more neutral stimulus. Similarly, the inclusion of certain adjectives or adverbs might significantly influence a person's responses.

This suggestibility is, of course, not confined to these exercises. Social psychologists demonstrated many years ago that simply introducing words such as warm or cold into the introductory descriptions of a person has a significant effect on subjects' responses (Kelley, 1950). However, in the relaxed state normally induced by guided imagery, subjects are even more suggestible than usual, and so even greater care must be taken to present the stimulus material in a totally neutral way. The potential dangers of suggestibility have been highlighted recently by the widespread publicity surrounding what is referred to as False Memory Syndrome. This alleges that false memories of childhood sexual abuse have been implanted (in some cases unintentionally and in others quite deliberately) in many clients during therapy, with dire consequences. Indeed, it is because confabulation is recognized as a common feature of hypnosis that evidence obtained in this way is inadmissible in British courts of law.

Incidental detail, unwittingly introduced by the guide when using imagery, may produce alarming effects. When experimenting with imagery to induce relaxation, the author suggested quite unintentionally to subjects that they would feel their legs become progressively tight, tired and heavy as they descended a long flight of stairs, only to discover that many of those who participated subsequently experienced pain in their legs for days afterwards. The only way in which these incidental contaminating features can be controlled for and eliminated is by rigorous standardization of both the stimulus materials and the mode of presentation, which inevitably means testing them in repeated trials with large numbers of subjects.

It is not only the words used in presenting imagery exercises that need to be carefully chosen, so too does the mode of speech or style of delivery. This is equally important whether material is being presented by one individual to another, to a group, or when making an audio-tape for oneself. Any tendency towards theatrical or dramatic delivery should be avoided because by so doing one effectively tells a story or creates the drama, rather than encouraging the individual to do so, and as such this constitutes a form of direction. On the other hand a flat monotone, rather than being relaxing or 'hypnotic' as some people suppose, is likely to have quite the opposite effect, giving rise to irritation and increased tension or sleep. The presenter should aim to speak in such a way that he or she does not 'get in the way' of the imagery process, rather than actively trying to facilitate it. This requires reasonably fluent delivery and a clear, calm, confident voice that is even in tone, without exaggerated emphasis, and smooth in pace.

Alternation of pitch, volume and pace is to be avoided:

> A good masseur knows that the client's mind tends to move at the pace of his hands, so when he wants the client to relax deeply, he starts at a medium speed and gradually moves more and more slowly. He avoids making any sudden or unexpected moves. The same principle applies to using our voices to create the deep relaxation in which imagery most easily arises. And again, the rhythm we work with is important (Macbeth, 1991, p. 24).

The pace of delivery will depend to some extent on the nature of the exercise and whether it is being presented to an individual or a group. If the exercise contains various suggestions or questions, then a pause after each is desirable so that the person may respond to them. When working with an individual who is answering directly or relating the experience aloud as it unfolds, this presents few problems. When the individual's responses are to be related after the exercise, or when more than one person is simultaneously engaged in the exercise, this is less straightforward. Inevitably the pace will be suitable for some, but either too fast or too slow for others. Achieving the modal pace (that which is appropriate to the majority) comes only with experience.

It may be thought that a very slow pace would accommodate most people. However, the ordinary time sense is altered during relaxation and imagery because mental events are not organized and processed sequentially but simultaneously. Events therefore do not unfold over time as they appear to ordinarily, but more or less instantaneously. Accordingly, relatively little time needs to be given to them, and when presentation of stimulus material is too slow respondents tend to become frustrated and irritated, or fall asleep.

The greatest temptation, however, is for the person guiding the imagery material to do so too quickly, especially if he or she has presented it on countless occasions. The time which passes in a flash for the imager may seem endless to the guide. For those with this tendency it is advisable to standardize the procedure, timing pauses with a watch if necessary.

Misguided interpretation

Whereas guided imagery exercises should be standardized so as to minimize the covert influence of the guide on an individual's responses, interpretation of the resulting images should be unstandardized and not guided by any dogma. Just as many guides believe that the symbolic elements of imagery which have been of personal value to them will be of universal validity, so they often assume that the specific personal meanings, insights and effects evoked by these elements will necessarily be generated in others. This results in this essentially subjective and idiosyncratic construct system becoming the definitive interpretive framework for the subjective experiences of others. Personal subjective interpretations of images are thus expressed as universal truths.

In this way, many guides perpetuate the fallacy given credence by Freud that they are 'expert' in the interpretation of images produced in dreams, fantasy, day-dreams and reverie. However (and this cannot be emphasized enough) this is simply not the case. As Jung indicated, although a person's imagery may have certain universal features, it represents nonetheless the unique symbolic language or representational system of the individual, which he or she must learn to translate and understand. Accordingly, the interpretation of a person's imagery by another, however, 'expert', will reveal only the features of the symbolic language of the latter, rather than that of their subject, and as such may be highly misleading. Accordingly, all such guidance is fundamentally misguidance. Not only can the guide mislead others, but also him- or herself, for as Von Franz (1975) has noted, such guidance can seduce the guide into what she terms 'the pride of the shaman', an evil warned against in primitive myths. Furthermore, she claims, it robs the individual of what is needed most, free inner responsibility.

It is essential, therefore, that individuals are encouraged to explore their own symbolic vocabulary, its meanings and usage. Much as they might discern the meaning of an unknown or unusual word or code. This can be done by examining its context, other available clues, similar sounding words, and patterns of usage, the associations it evokes, and attempting to identify its components in foreign or ancient languages. In this way individuals become expert in their own use of symbols. If they work with others in this enterprise they should ensure that the personal meaning of symbols is not lost in its translation by them.

WORKING WITH OTHERS

Other people, whether therapists, writers or friends, can have a valuable role in assisting people to understand their personal imagery. This can be done in a number of ways, such as helping people to explore their feelings and responses to imagery, and the associations it conjures for them. These may be verbalized, as favoured by Freud and his followers; or externalized through painting, drawing and other artwork, as advocated by Jung, and more recently by the Simontons and Elisabeth Kubler-Ross; expressed through drama, in the manner of Perls and Moreno; or by story telling (Roet, 1988). They can also amplify a person's responses to imagery by expressing the associations and responses the person's images and responses elicit in them, or by pointing to similar symbols and meanings in mythology and esoteric traditions, as did Jung, and making suggestions as to possible meanings.

Cousins (1981a) has indicated that the doctor is the greatest placebo and more effective than any medicine. This is undoubtedly true in relation to imagery. Research (Paul and Trimble, 1970; Tamez, Moore and Brown, 1978) has indicated that relaxation and imagery are more effective when live, rather than taped, instruction is received, for reasons that remain unclear. However, as Laing (1991) observed, 'treatment is not pills, it is the way we treat people; the way we attend to them'. Indeed, the term 'therapist' derives from the Greek *therapeia* meaning attendance. In the true sense of the word, therefore, it is the attention or assistance given to individuals and the significance of their imagery that constitutes 'therapy'. Irrespective of whether this is provided by a friend, acquaintance, qualified therapist or other trained professional, they should possess certain qualities.

They must be a willing and capable listener. This is not simply a matter of hearing what the person has to relate about his or her images and responses to them. It requires that an attempt be made to understand the nature of the experience, without direction, interpretation, criticism, ridicule, voyeurism or vicarious interest. The listener must be fully accepting of and open to the other's experience, genuinely supportive of the person in his or her exploration of it, open to the responses and associations the person's imagery evokes in him- or herself, and willing to share these without interpreting or theorizing about them. The listener must also be sensitive to and able to cope with the emotional reactions elicited by the person's imagery, allowing rather than suppressing or denying them.

It might be supposed that these qualities are generally to be found in those persons who offer themselves as guides, in psychotherapy or elsewhere. Regrettably this is no more the case than it is true that these qualities are possessed by all doctors and other health-care professionals, whose qualifications may be essentially intellectual rather than interpersonal.

Jourard (1971) has observed that many doctors, psychiatrists, therapists and counsellors are attracted to their professions not because of their desire to attend to others so much as to have others give attention to them. Not surprisingly therefore many 'therapists' have aspirations to power and dominance, authoritarian personalities, and more than their fair share of egotism and self-righteousness. So, just as there are doctors who do not listen and who rush into hasty and often unjustified diagnoses, there are 'therapists' and would-be therapists who do likewise. Moreover, just as there are some physicians who make hasty, ill-considered and inappropriate prescriptions for patients, or do not follow up treatment, so there are 'guides' who merely present clients with inappropriate guided imagery exercises without any systematic attempt to help people understand their responses to them, or to monitor effects. Giving people time and space to reflect on, and talk through their experiences is very important, because this is how insight is achieved. Not uncommonly, however, courses and workshops on guided imagery involve little more than the guide presenting a series of exercises without giving participants time to talk these through, much less discern their meaning and personal significance.

ANAPHYLAXIS

It should be appreciated that just as the body sometimes shows an extreme sensitivity to certain injected or ingested substances, so too individuals may experience a similar shock reaction to prescribed images or the insights they produce. Adverse reactions to images such as anxiety, fear, shock and panic can occur, although severe reactions are uncommon. Where they occur it is because the person's ordinary defences have been relaxed and issues usually repressed suddenly impinge on consciousness. This intrusion may be experienced psychically in much the way the sting of an insect might be experienced physically, and the person will often react accordingly. Hence a woman who participated in an imagery study group led by the author, experienced an intense shock reaction when undertaking an imagery-augmented relaxation procedure for the first time. Subsequently it transpired that she had considered herself to have dealt successfully with the issues underlying her long psychiatric history, until they resurfaced in the exercise. Her shock was a reaction, not only to the realization that these had not been resolved, but also to the fact that the only way she could pretend to herself that they had been was by maintaining a hypertense state; a defence which required only minimal relaxation to be breached.

Just as anaphylactic shock requires immediate treatment, so these reactions must be attended to directly, rather than ignored or dismissed. Recognizing signs of distress, prior to, during and after imagework, and attending to them, whether on a one-to-one or group basis, requires sensitivity and perceptiveness, and is often the most important feature of therapy. As has been noted previously, the Simontons recommend that cancer patients are helped to confront their fears directly. They argue that suppressed fears invariably constitute a greater threat to health and survival than the malignancy itself. Accordingly, to collude with a person in suppressing or dismissing the darker emotions and aspects of the self is likely to do more harm than good. They insist that helping a person to confront their fears, feelings of hopelessness, helplessness, despair and lack of self-control is a necessary step in the direction of health, recovery, greater vitality and improved quality of life. Once fear is reduced it is easier for people to develop a more positive expectancy, which not only results in further fear reduction but may also be a significant feature in cancer regression. Dossey (1982) also considers the panic, anxiety, depression and resignation associated with terminal illness to be in itself a malignant 'coping style' (a cancer which eats away at a person and should be dealt with as promptly as physical components of disease). Similarly, Jung considered that repression of the 'shocking' features of the self, when potentially painful or dangerous thoughts, desires and feelings are excluded from consciousness, leads to one-sided development of the personality rather than wholesome or healthy development, and that these features should be confronted.

PERSISTENT PROBLEMS

Treatment insensitivity

In contrast to those people in whom imagery produces powerful effects, there are those who insist that it does not work for them and is ineffective because their mind becomes 'blank' when they attempt to use it. In some instances this arises simply because they give insufficient time for imagery to develop and give up when an instantaneous reaction fails to occur. A similar reaction can be noted in relation to most treatments. Some people expect instant cure or recovery, without any effort or persistence on their own part. Such people frequently fail to complete a course of treatment.

While this response may be an indication of resistance, it may result from enthusiasm and impatience. Some people who wish to use imagery for self-healing are desperate to achieve results, and this factor needs to be recognized. In some instances the mind remains 'blank' because the person tries too hard to produce imagery, thereby creating tension rather than the relaxed state in which imagery is most easily and spontaneously produced. As with all other responses to imagery, awareness and close examination of tendencies such as impatience and/or trying too hard, and consideration of the ways in which they may contribute to a person's ills is to be encouraged.

Commonly, individuals fail to produce imagery because their rational, logical, verbal mind remains over-active and dominant. Relaxation procedures are usually effective in overcoming this difficulty, although for some individuals this occurs only slowly over time, with repetition and practice. An effective guide will, however, encourage an individual to explore this trait and to consider its possible implications for personal well-being, health and illness.

Received wisdom

While there is a great deal of truth in Ram Dass' assertion that 'you only get as high as your therapist', ultimately, the user or recipient of treatment the individual patient, or 'impatient', as the case may be, determines the effectiveness of guided imagery. Many of the anxieties and negative attitudes and beliefs which inhibit his or her use of guided imagery can be overcome or greatly reduced when adequate guidance and reassurance are provided. However, in the absence of adequate guidance many people who might otherwise derive great benefits from imagery do not continue in their attempts to do so. Even people who have achieved quite startling results with imagery during a course of therapy or supervised exercises, fail to continue with them when guidance is no longer available. A case in point is a woman who over a series of imagery exercises guided by the author achieved an amelioration in her hypertensive condition so dramatic that her consultant physician initially attributed the significant decrease in blood pressure to mis-reading of test results. Yet although this lowered blood pressure was sustained throughout the period she attended workshops and practised the recommended 'homework' exercises, she discontinued the exercises almost immediately each course ended, with the result that her blood pressure increased again. Indeed her imagery revealed that the problems underlying her medical condition, which generated high levels of anxiety and resulting tension, included very low self-esteem, lack of self-confidence, a belief that she could not achieve anything on her own, and a consequent over-dependence and reliance on others. She could therefore get on 'well', quite literally, only when 'doing as she was told'.

Physical and psychological withdrawal effects from imagery do occur, especially when people are using imagery in the alleviation of stress, stress-related, and stressful conditions. The Simontons (Simonton and Simonton, 1975) report that most cancer patients do not relax, and when asked to visualize usually do not do so in a positive way. Moreover, they found that the positive attitude of many patients in their initial investigation only lasted during the treatment programme. After that they reverted to negative attitudes, viewing themselves as victims of illness and unable personally to do anything to help themselves get well.

These experiences highlight the artificiality of the therapeutic situation, and the fact that results achieved therein do not necessarily translate to ordinary life where there are competing demands, pressures and activities; and often a lack of support and affirmation for the individual. Simonton and Simonton (1975) have emphasized the importance of the family belief system in encouraging or undermining effective outcomes; indicating that without support little can be achieved. Abundant research has since confirmed that social support is essential to health (Sarason, Sarason and Pierce, 1988, 1990). Lack of support by family and friends may also deter people from embarking on, or continuing with, exercises on their own. For this reason it is advisable to recommend individuals to practice the exercises with one or more friends. Small informal groups can be a very effective means of establishing a support network.

Factors such as those noted above, rather than lack of interest, enthusiasm or discipline, are likely to prevent people taking time to familiarize themselves with relevant procedures, or to put time aside each day for image work. As is the case with conventional medicines therefore, some people will fail to follow the full course of treatment, recommendations for use, or correct procedures. These user variables will tend to produce ineffective results, irrespective of the adequacy of the prescribed formulae and the guidance and support provided. Ultimately therefore, the therapeutic effectiveness of imagery depends on the individual user, and this has to be borne in mind in every instance where imagery is recommended or prescribed. As a result, outcomes will be extremely variable. Nevertheless, the author's conclusions, based on extensive experience of working with imagery in many contexts and applications, and with a great number and diversity of people, supports the observation of Anatole France that 'to accomplish great things we must not only act, but also dream'.

References

Abse, D.W. *et al.* (1974) Personality and behavioural characteristics of lung cancer patients. *J. Psychosomatic Res.*, **18**, 101–113.

Achterberg, J. (1984) Imagery and medicine: Psychophysiological speculations. *J. Mental Imagery*, **8**, 1–13.

Achterberg, J. (1985) *Imagery in Healing: Shamanism and Modern Medicine*. Routledge and Kegan Paul, London.

Achterberg, J. and Lawlis, G.F. (1978) *Imagery of Cancer*. Institute for Personality and Ability Testing, Champaign, Illinois.

Achterberg, J. and Lawlis, G.F. (1979) A canonical analysis of blood chemistry variables related to psychological measures of cancer patients. *Multivariate Exp. Clin. Res.*, **3**, 107–22.

Achterberg, J., Simonton, O.C. and Simonton, S.M. (1977) Psychology of the exceptional cancer patient: A description of patients who outlive predicted life expectancies. *Psychotherapy: Theory Res. Practice*, **14**, 416–22.

Ader, R. (ed.) (1981) *Psychoneuroimmunology*. Academic Press, New York.

Ader, R. (1983) Developmental psychoneuroimmunology. *Dev. Psychobiol*, **16** (4), 251–67.

Ader, R. (1985) Behaviourally conditioned modulation of immunity, in *Neural Modulation of Immunity*, (eds R. Guillemin, M. Cohn and A. Melnechuk), Raven Press, New York, pp. 56–66.

Ader, R. and Cohen, N. (1975) Behaviourally conditioned immunosuppression. *Psychosomatic Med.*, **37**, 333–40.

Ader, R. and Cohen, N. (1981) Conditioned immunopharmacologic effects, in *Psychoneuroimmunology*, (ed. R. Ader), Academic Press, New York, pp. 281–319.

Ahsen, A. (1978) Eidetics: Neural experiential growth potential for the treatment of accident traumas, debilitating stress conditions and chronic emotional blocking. *J. Mental Imagery*, **2**, 1–22.

Alvarez, A. (1989) Stressful life events and the recurrence of breast cancer in women. Reported in Medicine Now, BBC Radio 4, 15 February.

Amkraut, A.A., Solomon, G.F. and Kraemer, H.C. (1971) Stress, early experience and adjuvant induced arthritis in the rat. *Psychosomatic Med.*, **33**, 203–14.

Amussat, J.Z. (1854) *Quelques Reflections sur la Credibility du Cancer*. Paris.

Anand, B.K., Chhina, G.S. and Singh, B. (1961a) Studies on Shri Ramananda Yogi during his stay in an airtight box. *Indian J. Med. Res.*, **49**, 82–9.

Anand, B.K., Chhina, G.S. and Singh, B. (1961b) Some aspects of electroencephalographic studies in yogis. *Electroencephalography Clin. Neurophysiology*, **13**, 452–6.

Anderson, M. (1962) *The Unknowable Gurdjieff*. Routledge and Kegan Paul, London.

Anderson, M. (1969) *The Strange Necessity*. Horizon Press, New York.

Anderson, N. (1982) *Open Secrets: A Western Guide to Tibetan Buddhism*. Penguin, Harmondsworth.

Andrews, L. (1981) *Medicine Woman*. Harper & Row, San Francisco.

Anonymous (1985) Emotion and immunity. *Lancet*, **11**, 133–4.

Anonymous (1987) Depression, stress and immunity. *Lancet*, **27**, 1467–68.

Arabian, J.M. (1982) Imagery and Pavlovian heart rate decelerative conditioning. *Psychophysiology*, **19**, 286–93.

Arabian, J.M. and Furedy, J.J. (1983) Individual differences in imagery ability and Pavlovian heart rate decelerative conditioning. *Psychophysiology*, **20**, 325–31.

Arehart-Treichel, J. (1982) Pets: the health benefits. *Sci. News*, **121**, 220–4.

Arkow, P. (1984) *Dynamic Relationships in Practice: Animals in the Helping Professions*. Latham Foundation, Alameda, California.

Ashe, G. (1977) *The Ancient Wisdom*. MacMillan, London.

Asistent, N.M. with Duffy, P. (1991) *Why I Survive AIDS*. Simon and Schuster, New York.

Assagioli, R. (1965) *Psychosynthesis: A Collection of Basic Writings*. Viking, New York.

Assagioli, R. (1967) *Jung and Psychosynthesis*. Psychosynthesis Foundation, New York.

Assagioli, R. (1975) *Psychosynthesis*. Turnstone Press, Wellingborough.

Assagioli, R. (1991a) *Transpersonal Development*. Crucible, London.

Assagioli, R. (1991b) Psychosynthesis, in *The New Age: An Anthology of Essential Writings*, (ed. W. Bloom), Rider, London, pp. 118–24.

Bagchi, B.K. and Wenger, M.A. (1959) Electrophysiological correlates of some yoga exercises, in *Electroencephalography, Clinical Neurophysiology and Epilepsy, Vol.3 of First Congress of Neurological Sciences*, (eds L.van Bagaert and J. Radermecker), Pergamon, London.

Bahnson, C.B. (1969) Psychophysiological complementarity in malignancies: past work and future vistas. *Ann. New York Acad. Sci.*, **125**, 802–6.

Baigent, M., Leigh. R. and Lincoln, H. (1982) *The Holy Blood and The Holy Grail*. Cape, London.

Baltrusch, H.J.F. and Waltz, N. (1986) Early family attitudes and the stress process: a lifespan and personological model of host-tumor relationships, in *Cancer, Stress and Death*, (ed. S.B. Day), Plenum Medican, New York.

Bancroft, A. (1978) *Modern Mystics and Sages*. Paladin, London.

Bandler, R. and Grinder, J. (1975) *The Structure of Magic. Vol. I. Science and Behavior*. California Press, Palo Alto, California.

Barber, J. (1987) On not beating dead horses. *Br. J. Exp. Clin. Hypnosis*, **4**, 156–7.

Barber, T.X. (1961) Psychological aspects of hypnosis. *Psychological Bull.*, **58**, 390–419.

Barber, T.X. (1969) *Hypnosis: A Scientific Approach*. Van Nostrand, New York.

Barber, T.X., Spanos, N.P. and Chaves, J.F. (1974) *Hypnosis, Imagination and Human Potentialities*. Pergamon, New York.

Barber, T.X. (1978) Hypnosis, suggestions and psychosomatic phenomena: a new look from the standpoint of recent experimental studies. *Am. J. Clin. Hypnosis*, **21**, 13–27.

Barber, T.X., Chauncey, H.H. and Winer, R.A. (1964) Effects of hypnotic and non-hypnotic suggestion on parotid gland response to gustatory stimuli. *Psychosomatic Med.*, **26**, 374–80.

Bartrop, R.W. *et al.*, (1977) Depressed lymphocyte function after bereavement. *Lancet*, **1**, 834–6.

Bauer, R.M. and Craighead, W.E. (1979) Psychophysiological responses to the imagination of fearful and neutral situations: the effects of imagery instructions. *Behaviour Therapy*, **10**, 389–403.

Beach, F.A. (1948) *Hormones and Behaviour.* Harper, New York.

Beecher, H.K. (1955) The powerful placebo. *J. Am. Med. Assoc.*, **159**, 1602–6.

Bell, I.R. and Schwartz, G.E. (1975) Voluntary control and reactivity of human heart rate. *Psychophysiology*, **12**, 339–48.

Benson, H.D. *et al.*, (1974) Decreased blood pressure in pharmacologically treated hypertensive patients who regularly elicited the relaxation response. *Lancet*, 23 March, 289.

Benson, H.D. with Zlipper, M.Z. (1975) *The Relaxation Response.* Collins, London.

Bergman, R.L. (1973) A school for medicine men. *Am. J. Psychiatry*, **130**, 663–6.

Besant, A. (1899) *The Ancient Wisdom: An Outline of Theosophical Teachings.* 2nd ed. Theosophical Publishing Society: Aberdeen University Press, London.

Bertrand, L.D. and Spanos, N.P. (1989) Hypnosis: historical and social psychological aspects, in *Eastern and Western Approaches to Healing: Ancient Wisdom and Modern Knowledge*, (eds A.A. Sheikh and K.S. Sheikh), Wiley, New York, pp. 237-63.

Beveridge, W.I.B. (1957) *The Art of Scientific Investigation.* 3rd ed., Vintage, New York.

Binswanger, H. (1929) Beobachtungen an entspannten and versenkten Versuchspersonen: Ein Beitrag zu Moglichen Mechanismen der Konversionhysterie. *Nervenarzt*, **4**, 193.

Bishopric, M.J., Cohen, H.J. and Leftowitz, R.J. (1980) Beta-adrenergic receptors in lymphocyte subpopulations. *J. Allergy Clin. Immunol.*, **65**, 29-33.

Bisiach, E. *et al.*, (1981) Brain and conscious representation of outside reality. *Neuropsychologia*, **19**, 543–51.

Bisiach, E. and Luzatti, C. (1978) Unilateral neglect of representational space. *Cortex*, **14**, 129–33.

Bisiach, E., Luzatti, C. and Persni, D. (1979) Unilateral neglect, representational schema and consciousness. *Brain*, **102**, 609–18.

Blair, L. (1975) *Rhythms of Vision.* Croom Helm, London.

Blavatsky, H. (1888) *The Secret Doctrine: The Synthesis of Science, Religion and Philosophy, Vols. 1–3.* The Theosophical Publishing House, London.

Blizard, D.A., Cowings, P. and Miller, N.E. (1975) Visceral responses to opposite types of autogenic-training imagery. *Biol. Psychol.*, **4**, 49–55.

Bloom, W. (ed.) (1991) *The New Age: An Anthology of Essential Writings.* Rider, London.

Bloomfield, H., Cain, M. and Jaffe, R. (1975) *TM: Discovering Inner Energy and Overcoming Stress.* Delacorte Press, New York.

Blumberg, E.M., West, P.M. and Ellis, F.W. (1954) A possible relationship between psychological factors and human cancer. *Psychosomatic Med.*, **16**, 277–86.

Blythe, P. (1979) Hypnosis, in *A Visual Encyclopaedia of Unconventional Medicine*, (ed. A. Hill), London: New English Library, London, pp. 188–9.

Boersma, F.J. and Houghton, A.A. (1990) Dreamwork with a cancer patient: the emergence of transpersonal healing. *Med. Hypnoanalysis J.*, March, 3–23.

Bohm, D. (1980) *Wholeness and the Implicate Order*. Routledge and Kegan Paul, London.

Booker, H.E., Rubow, R.T. and Coleman, P.J. (1969) Simplified feedback in neuromuscular training: An automated approach using electromyographic signals. *Arch. Physical Med. Rehabilitation*, 615–21.

Boot, K. (1993) A–Z of beliefs: Gnosticism. *Observer*, 18 July, 49.

Borysenko, M. (1987) Area Review: psychoneuroimmunology. *Ann. Behav. Med.*, **9**, 3–10.

Borysenko, M. and Borysenko, J. (1982) Stress, behavior and immunity: animal models and mediating mechanisms. *Gen. Hosp. Psychiatry*, **4**, 59–67.

Boudreau, L. (1972) Transcendental meditation and yoga as reciprocal inhibitors. *J. Behav. Ther. Exp. Psychiatry*, **3**, 97–8.

Bovberg, D., Ader, R. and Cohen, N. (1984) Acquisition and extinction of conditioned suppression of a graft-vs-host response in the rat. *J. Imunol.*, **132**, 111–3.

Bowers, K.S. (1976) *Hypnosis for the Seriously Curious*. Brooks/Cole, Monterey, California.

Bradley, B. and McCanne, T. (1981) Autonomic responses to stress; the effects of progressive relaxation, the relaxation response and the expectancy of relief. *Biofeedback Self Regulation*, **6**, 235–51.

Branthwaite, J.A. and Cooper, P. (1989) Psychology and Market Research, in *The Applied Psychologist*, (eds J. Hartley and J.A. Branthwaite), Open University Press, Milton Keynes.

Brayton, A.R. and Brain, P.F. (1975) Effects of differential housing and glucocorticoid administration on immune responses to sheep red blood cells in albino TO strain mice. *J. Endocrinol.*, **54** (1), 4–5.

Brener, J. and Kleinman, R.A. (1970) Learned control of descreases in systolic blood pressure. *Nature*, **26**, 1063.

Breznitz, S. (1984) *The Denial of Stress*. International Universities Press, New York.

British Broadcasting Corporation (1994) Death Wish. Horizon, BBC2, 7 February.

Broadhead, W.E. *et al.* (1983) The epidemiological evidence for a relationship between social support and health. *Am. J. Epidemiol.*, **117**, 5, 521–37.

Brohn, P. (1986) *Gentle Giants*. Century, London.

Bryden, M.P. and Ley, R.G. (1983) Right hemisphere involvement in imagery and affect, in *Cognitive processing in the right hemisphere*, (ed. E. Perecman), Academic Press, New York.

Buckley, L. (1993) *The Shamanic Path to Mental Health*. Paper presented at The Third Annual Conference: The Promotion of Mental Health European Conference, Botanical Gardens, Birmingham, England, 6–8 September.

Burish, T.G. and Lyles, J.N. (1981) Effects of relaxation training in reducing adverse reactions to cancer chemotherapy. *J. Behavioural Med.*, **4**, 65–78.

Bulloch, K. and Moore, R.Y. (1981) Innervation of the thymus gland by brainstem and spinal cord in mouse and rat. *Am. J. Anat.*, **162**, 157–66.

Burrows, J. (1783) *A Practical Essay on Cancer*. London.

Butler, W.E. (1982) *Magic: Its Ritual, Power and Purpose*. The Aquarian Press, Wellingborough, Northants.

Cannon, W.B. (1929) *Bodily Changes in Pain, Hunger, Fear and Rage*. 2nd edn., Appleton, New York.

Canter, A. (1972) Changes in mood during incubation of acute febrile disease and the effects of pre-exposure psychological status. *Psychosomatic Med.*, **34**, 424–5.

Capra, F. (1976) *The Tao of Physics*. Fontana, London.

Capra, F. (1982a) *The Turning Point: Science, Society and the Rising Culture*. Wildwood House, London.

Capra, F. (1982b) Foreword to Dossey, L. *Space, Time and Medicine*. Shambhala, Boulder, Colorado.

Carroll, D., Baker, J. and Preston, M. (1979) Individual differences in normal imaging and the voluntary control of heart rate. *Br. J. Psychol.*, **70**, 39–49.

Carroll, D., Marzillier, J.S. and Merian, S. (1982) Psychophysiological changes accompanying different types of arousing and relaxing imagery. *Psychophysiology*, **19**, 75–82.

Carson, D.A. (1993) Apoptosis and disease. *Lancet*, **341**, 1251–4.

Castaneda, C. (1973) *A Separate Reality*. Penguin, Harmondsworth.

Castaneda, C. (1975) *Journey to Ixtlan*. Penguin, Harmondsworth.

Castaneda, C. (1976) *Tales of Power*. Penguin, Harmondsworth.

Castaneda, C. (1978) *The Second Ring of Power*. Penguin, Harmondsworth.

Castaneda, C. (1982) *The Eagle's Gift*. Penguin, Harmondsworth.

Castaneda, C. (1984) *The Power Within*. Black Swan Books, London.

Castaneda, C. (1988) *The Power of Silence*. Black Swan Books, Transworld.

Castaneda, C. (1993) *The Art of Dreaming*. The Aquarian Press, London.

Cautela, J. (1967) Covert desensitization. *Psychological Rep.*, **20**, 459–68.

Cautela, J.R. (1993) *Covert Conditioning Casebook*. Brooks/Cole, New York.

Chaves, J.F. (1980) Hypnotic control of surgical bleeding. Paper presented at the Annual meeting of the Am. Psychological Association, Montreal, in *Imagery and Healing*, (ed. A.A. Sheikh), Baywood, Farmingdale, New York, pp. 65–158.

Chertok, L. (1969) *The Evolution of Research into Hypotheses in Psychophysiological Mechanisms of Hypnosis*. Springer Verlag, New York.

Chertok, L. (1981) *Sense and Nonsense in Psychotherapy: The Challenge of Hypnosis*. Pergamon Press, Oxford.

Chevalier, G. (1976) *The Sacred Magician: A Ceremonial Diary*. Paladin, London.

Clark, N. and Fraser, S.T. (1987) *The Gestalt Approach*, 2nd edn., Roffey Park Management College, Horsham.

Clarkson, P. and MacKewn, J. (1993) *Fritz Perls*, Sage, London.

Clarkson, P. and Shaw, P. (1992) Human relationships at work – the place of counselling skills and consulting skills and services in organizations. *J. Assoc. Manage. Education Dev.*, **23**, 18–29.

Clifford, T. (1984) *Tibetan Buddhist Medicine and Psychiatry*. Samuel Weiser, New York.

Coates, T.J. and Greenblatt, R.M. (1986), Behavioural change using intervention at the community level, in *Sexually Transmitted Disease*, (ed. K.K. Holmes), McGraw-Hill, New York.

Colegrave, S. (1979) *The Spirit of the Valley: Androgyny and Chinese Thought*. Virago, London.

Cooper, L.A. and Shepard, R.N. (1973) Chronometric studies of the rotation of mental images, in *Visual Information Processing*, (ed. W.G. Chase), Academic Press, New York.

Cooper, R.N. (1975) Mental rotation of random two-dimensional shapes. *Cognitive Psychology*, **7**, 20–43.

Cooper, M. and Aygen, M. (1978) Effect of meditation on blood cholesterol and blood pressure. *J. Israel Med. Assoc.*, **95**, 2.

Cooper, G., Cooper, R. and Eaker, L. (1988) *Living With Stress.* Penguin, Harmondsworth.

Cosgrove, M.P. (1982) *Psychology Gone Awry: Four Psychological World Views.* Inter-Varsity Press, Leicester.

Cousins, N. (1981a) *Anatomy of an Illness as perceived by the Patient: Reflections on Healing and Regeneration.* Bantam, London.

Cousins, N. (1981b) *Human Options.* W.W.Norton, New York.

Craig, K.D. (1968) Physiological arousal as a function of imagined, vicarious and direct stress experience. *J. Abnormal Psychology*, **73**, 513–20.

Crowther, J.H. (1983) Stress management training and relaxation imagery in the treatment of essential hypertension. *J. Behavioural Med.*, **6**, 169–87.

Dass, R. (1978) *Journey of Awakening: A Meditator's Guidebook.* Hanuman Foundation, New York.

Dattore, P.J., Schontz, F.C. and Coyne, L. (1980) Premorbid personality differentiation of cancer and non-cancer group: A test of the hypothesis of cancer proneness. *J. Consulting Clin. Psychology*, **48**, 388–94.

Davis, D.E. and Read, C.P. (1958) Effect of behavior on development of resistance in trichinosis. *Proc. Soc. Exp. Biol. Med.*, **99**, 269–72.

Day, H. (1953) *The Study and Practice of Yoga.* Thorsons Publishing, London.

De Mille, R. (1978) *Castaneda's Journey.* Abacus, London.

De Mille, R. (ed.) (1980) *The Don Juan Papers: More Castaneda Controversies.* Ross Erikson, Santa Barbara.

Derogatis, L., Abeloff, M. and Melisarotos, N. (1979) Psychological coping mechanisms and survival time in metastatic breast cancer. *J. Am. Med. Assoc.*, **242**, 1504–8.

Desoille, R. (1945) *The Waking Dream in Psychotherapy: An essay on the regulatory function of the collective unconscious (La Reveille eveille en psychotherapie).* Universitaire, Paris.

Desoille, R. (1965) *The Directed Daydream.* Psychosynthesis Research Foundation, New York.

Dillon, K.M., Minchoff, B. and Baker, K.H. (1985) Positive emotional states and enhancement of the immune system. *Int. J. Psychiatry Med.*, **15**, 13–17.

Dirks, J.F., Robinson, S.K. and Dirks, D.L. (1981) Alexithymia and the psychomaintenance of bronchial asthma. *Psychotherapy and Psychosomatics*, **36**, 63–71.

Dohrenwend, B.S. (1974) *Stressful Life Events, Their Nature and Effects.* Wiley, New York.

Donovan, M. (1980) Relaxation with guided imagery: a useful technique. *Cancer Nursing*, **3**, 27–32.

Dorian, B.J. *et al.* (1982) Aberrations in lymphocyte subpopulations and functions during psychological stress. *Clin. Exp. Immunol.*, **50**, 132–8.

Dossey, L. (1982) *Space, Time and Medicine.* Shambhala, Boston.

Dossey, L. (1989) The importance of modern physics for modern medicine, in *Eastern and Western Approaches to Healing: Ancient Wisdom and Modern Knowledge*, (eds A.A. Sheikh and K.S. Sheikh), Wiley, Chichester, pp. 395–423

Dostalek, C. (1987) The empirical and experimental foundation of yoga therapy, in *The Art of Survival: A Guide to Yoga Therapy*, (eds D.M. Gharote and M. Lockhart), Unwin Hyman, London.

Drummond, P., White, K. and Ashton, R. (1978) Imagery vividness affects habituation rate. *Psychophysiotherapy*, **15**, 193–5.

Drury, N. (1978) *Don Juan, Mescalito and Modern magic: A Mythology of Inner Space*. Routledge and Kegan Paul, London.

Drury, N. (1979) *Inner Visions: explorations in magical consciousness*. Routledge and Kegan Paul, London.

Drury, N. (1987) *The Shaman and The Magician: journeys between the worlds*. Penguin, Harmondsworth.

Drury, N. (1987) *The Occult Experience*. Robert Hale, London.

Drury, N. (1991) *The Elements of Shamanism*. Element Books, Shaftesbury.

Dugan, M. and Sheridan, C. (1976) Effects of instructed imagery on temperature of the hands. *Perceptual and Motor Skills*, **42**, 14.

Duncker, K. (1945) On problem solving. *Psychological Monographs*, **58** (5), No. 270, 1–111.

Edelstein, E.J. and Edelstein, L. (1945) *Asclepius: A collection and interpretation of the testimonies*. Johns Hopkins University Press, Baltimore, Maryland.

Edwards, E.A. and Dean, L.M. (1977) Effects of crowding of mice on humoral antibody formation and protection of lethal antigenic challenge. *Psychosomatic Med.*, **39**, 19–24.

Edwards, E.A. *et al.* (1980) Antibody response to bovine serum albumin in mice: the effects of psychosocial environmental change. *Proc. Soc. Exp. Biol. Med.*, **164**, 478–81.

Edwards, G. (1991) *Living Magically: A New Vision of reality*. Piatkus, London.

Eiff, A. and Jorgens, H. (1961) Die Spindelelrregbarkeit beim autogenem training, in Proceedings of the Third International Congress on Psychiatry, Montreal.

Elder, S.T. (1977) Apparatus and procedure for training subjects to control blood pressure. *Psychophysiology*, **14**, 68.

Eliade, M. (1989) *Shamanism: Archaic Techniques of Ecstasy*. (Translated from the French by W.R. Trask, Penguin, Harmondsworth. First published 1964), Pantheon Bollingen Foundation, New York.

Ellenberger, H.H. (1970) *The Discovery of the Unconscious*. Basic Books, New York.

Engel, B.T. (1972) Operant conditioning of cardiac functioning. *Psychophysiology*, **9**, 161.

Engel. B.T. (1979) Behavioural applications in the treatment of patients with cardiovascular disorders, in *Biofeedback: Principles and Practices for Clinicians*, (ed. J.V. Basmajian), Williamns and Wilkins, Baltimore, Maryland.

Epes-Brown, J. (1985) North American Indian Religions, in *A Handbook of Living Religions*, (ed. J.R. Hinnells), Penguin, Harmondsworth, pp. 392–411.

Erhlichman, H. and Barrett, J. (1983) Right hemisphere specialization for mental imagery: a review of evidence. *Brain and Cognition*, **2**, 52.

Erickson, M.H. (1959) Hypnosis in painful terminal illness. *Am. J. Clin. Hypnosis*, **2**, 117–122, 95–101.

Ernst, S. and Goodison, L. (1981) *In Your Own Hands: A book of self-help therapy*. Women's Press, london.

Evan, G.I. (1993) The role of c-myc in cell growth. *Current Opinion Genetics Dev.*, **3**, 26.

Evans, S. (1926) *A Psychological Study of Cancer*. Dodd Mead, New York.

Evans-Wentz, W.Y. (1967) *Tibetan Yoga and Secret Doctrines*. Oxford University Press, London.

Evans-Wentz, W.Y. (1976) *The Tibetan Book of the Dead*. Oxford University Press, Oxford.

Fagan, J. and Shepherd, I.L. (1971) *Gestalt Therapy Now: Theory/ Technique/Applications*. Harper & Row, New York.

Farah, M.J. (1984) The neurological basis of mental imagery: a componential analysis. *Cognition*, **18**, 245–72.

Farah, M.J. (1986) The laterality of mental image generation: a test with normal subjects. *Neuropsychologia*, **24**, 541–51.

Farah, M.J. *et al.* (1985) A left hemisphere basis for visual mental imagery? *Neuropsychologia*, **23**, 115–8.

Farah, M.J. (1989a) Mechanisms of imagery–perception interaction. *J. Exp. Psychology: Human Perception and Performance*, **15**, 203–11.

Farah, M.J. (1989b) The neuropsychology of mental imagery, in *Neuropsychology of Visual Perception*, (ed. J.W. Brown), Lawrence Erlbaum Associates, Hillsdale, New Jersey, pp. 183–201.

Ferguson, M. (1983) *The Aquarian Conspiracy: Personal and Social Transformation in the 1980s*. Paladin, London.

Feynman, R. (1993) No ordinary genius: A portrait of Richard Feynman. BBC Horizon, 1 February.

Finke, R.A. (1989) *Principles of Mental Imagery*. MIT Press, Cambridge, Massachusetts.

Fiore, N. (1974) Fighting cancer: one patient's perspective. *New England J. Med.*, **300**, 284.

Frankl, V.E. (1969) *The Doctor and the Soul*. Souvenir Press, London.

Frederking, W. (1948) Deep relaxation and symbolism. *Psyche*, **2**.

Fretigny, R. and Virel, A. (1968) *L'imagerie mentale*. Mont Blanc, Geneva.

Freedom Long, M. (1954) *The Secret Science Behind Miracles*. Huna Research Publications, Vista, California.

Friedmann, E. *et al.* (1982) Animal companions and one-year survival of patients after discharge from a coronary care unit. *California Veterinarian*, **8**, 45–50.

Friedmann, E. *et al.* (1983) Social interaction and blood pressure: influence of animal companions. *J. Nervous and Mental Diseases*, **171** (8), 461–5.

Friedman, M. and Rosenman, R.H. (1974) *Type A Behaviour and Your Heart*. Alfred A Knopf, New York.

Fromm, E. (1951) *Psychoanalysis and Religion*. Gollancz, London.

Fromm, E. (1980) *Greatness and Limitations of Freud's Thought*. Cape, London.

Furedy, J.J. and Klajner, F. (1978) Imaginational Pavlovian conditioning of large-magnitude cardiac decelerations wit tilt as UCS. *Psychophysiology*, **15**, 538–48.

Furedy, J.J. and Poulos, C.X. (1976) Heart-rate decelerative Pavlovian conditioning with tilt as UCS: towards behavioural control of cardiac dysfunction. *Biol. Psychol.*, **4**, 93–106.

Gage, M.J. (1893) *Women, Church and State*. Chicago, Illinois.

Gallegos, E.S. (1983) Animal imagery, the chakra system and psychotherapy. *J. Transpersonal Psychology*, **15** (2), 125–36.

Gallegos, E.S. (1989) *The Personal Totem Pole: Animal Imagery, the Chakras and Psychotherapy*. Moon Bear Press, Santa Fe.

Gallegos, E.S. (1993) *Animals of the Four Windows: Integrating, Sensing, Feeling and Imagery*. Bear and Co, Santa Fe.

Galton, F. (1883) *Inquiries into Human Faculty and its Development*. MacMillan, London.

Ganster, D.C. and Victor, B. (1988) The impact of social support on mental and physical health. *Br. J. Med. Psychology*, **61**, 17–36.

Gawain, S. (1985) *Creative Visualization*. Bantam, New York.

Gawain, S. and King, L. (1988) *Living in the Light*. Eden Grove, London.

Gellatly, A. (1986) How memory skills can be improved, In (ed. A. Gellatly), *The Skilful Mind: An Introduction to Cognitive Psychology*, Open University Press, Milton Keynes.

Geschwind, N. and Behan, P. (1982) Left-handedness: Association with immune disease, migraine and developmental learning disorder. *Proc. Natl. Acad. Sci. USA*, **79**, 5097–100

Ghiselin, B. (1952) *The Creative Process*. New American Library, New York.

Gibran, K. (1978) *The Prophet*. Book Club Associates, London.

Gillespie, J. (1989) *Brave Heart*. Century, London.

Giovacchini, P.l. and Muslin, H. (1965) Ego equilibrium and cancer of the breast. *Psychosomatic Med.*, **27**, 524–32.

Glaser, R. *et al.* (1985a) Stress, loneliness and changes in herpes virus latency. *J. Behavioural Med.*, **8**, 249–60.

Glaser, R. *et al.* (1985b) Stress-related impairments in cellular immunity. *Psychiatric Res.*, **16**, 233–9.

Glouberman, D. (1989) *Life Choices and Life Changes Through Imagework*. Mandala, London.

Glusko, R.J. and Cooper, L.A. (1978) Spatial comprehension and comparison processes in verification tasks. *Cognitive Psychology*, **10**, 391–421.

Goodkin, K., Antoni, M.H. and Blaney, P.H. (1986) Stress and hopelessness in the promotion of cervical intraepithelial neoplasis to invasive squarous cell carcinoma of the cervix. *J. Psychosomatic Res.*, **30** (1), 67–76.

Gorczpynski, R.M., Macrae, S. and Kennedy, M. (1982) Conditioned immune response associated with allogeneic skin grafts in mice. *J. Immunology*, **129**, 704–9.

Gorman, P. and Kamiya, J. (1972) Voluntary control of stomach pH. Research note presented at Biofeedback Research Society Meeting, Boston, November.

Gorton, B. (1959) Autogenic Training. *Am. J. Clin. Hypnosis*, **2**, 31–41.

Gottschalk, L.A. (1974) Self-induced visual imagery, affect arousal and autonomic correlates. *Psychosomatics*, **15**, 166–9.

Graham, H. (1986) *The Human Face of Psychology: Humanistic Psychology in its Historical, Social and Cultural Context*. Open University Press, Milton Keynes.

Graham, H. (1990) *Time, Energy and the Psychology of Healing*. Jessica Kingsley, London.

Graham, H. (1992) *The Magic Shop: an imaginative guide to self-healing*. Rider, London.

Graham, H. (1995) *A Picture of Health: How to Use Guided Imagery for Self-healing and Personal Growth*. Piatkus, London.

Grassi, L. and Lodi, N. (1989) Early family relationships and parental losses among lung cancer patients. *New Trends Exp. Clin. Psychiatry*, **4**, 245–56.

Green, E.E. (1969) Voluntary control of inner states. *Psychophysiology*, **6**, 371.

Green, E.E. and Green, A.M. (1977) *Beyond Biofeedback*. Delacorte, New York.

Greene, A. and Miller, G. 1958 Psychological factors and reticloendothelial disease. *Psychosomatic Med.*, **20**, 124–44.

Greer, S., Morris, T. and Pettingdale, K.W. (1979) Psychological response to breast cancer: effect and outcome. *Lancet*, 2, 785–7.

Greer, S. and Watson, M. (1985) Towards a model of cancer: psychological considerations. *Social Sci. Med.*, **20** (8), 773–7.

Grof, S. (1979) *Realms of the Unconscious.* Souvenir Press, London.

Grof, S. (1985) *Beyond the Brain: birth, death and transcendence in psychotherapy.* SUNY Press, Albany.

Grof, S. (1992) *The Holotrophic Mind.* Harper, San Francisco.

Grossarth-Maticek, R., Bastians, J. and Kanazir, D.T. (1985) Psychosocial factors as strong predictors of mortality from cancer, ischaemic heart disease and stroke: the Yugoslav prospective study. *J. Psychosomatic Res.*, **29**, 167–76.

Grossberg, J. and Alf, E.F. (1984) Interaction with pet dogs: effect on human blood pressure. Presented at 92nd Annual Convention of the American Medical Association, Toronto, Canada.

Grossberg, J.M. and Wilson, K.M. (1968) Physiological changes accompanying the visualization of fearful and neutral situations. *J. Personality and Social Psychology*, **10**, 124–33.

Gunther, B. (1979) *Energy Ecstasy and Your Seven Vital Chakras.* 2nd edn., Guild of Tutors' Press, Los Angeles, California.

Gurdjieff, G. (1978) *Meetings With Remarkable Men.* Pan, London.

Gurdjieff, G. (1974) *Views From the Real World: the Early Talks of Gurdjieff.* Routledge and Kegan Paul, London.

Gurdjieff, G. (1976) *All And Everything: First Series – An Objectively Impartial Criticism of the Life of Man.* Routledge and Kegan Paul, London.

Guy, R. (1759) *An Essay on Scirrhous Tumours and Cancers.* J. and A. Churchill: The Welcome Historical Medical Library, London.

Hadamard, J. (1945) *The Psychology of Invention in the Mathematical Field.* Princeton University Press, Princeton, New Jersey.

Hall, H.R., Longo, S. and Dixon, R. (1981) Hypnosis and the immune system: the effect of hypnosis on T and B cell function. Paper presented at 33rd Annual Meeting of the Society for Clinical and Experimental Hypnosis, Portland, Oregon, reported by Hall, H.R. (1984).

Hall, H.R. (1984) Imagery and cancer, in *Imagination and Healing*, (ed. A.A. Sheikh), Baywood, Farmingdale, New York, pp. 159–69.

Hall, H.R. (1985) Hypnosis and the immune system: a review with implications for cancer and the psychology of healing. *Am. J. Clin. Hypnosis*, **25**, 92–103.

Hamachek, D.E. (1971) *Encounters With The Self.* Holt, Rhinehart and Winston, New York.

Haney, J.N. and Euse, F.J. (1976) Skin conductance and heart rate responses to neutral, positive and negative imagery: implications for covert behaviour therapy procedures. *Behaviour Therapy*, **7**, 494–503.

Happich, C. (1932) Das Bildenwusstsein als Ansatzstelle Psychischer behandlung. *Zbl. Psychoth.*, **5**, 663–7.

Happich, C. (1939) Symbolic consciousness and the creative situation. *Deutsch Med. Wschr.*, **2**

Happich, C. (1948) *Introduction to Meditation*, 3rd edn., E. Rother, Darmstadt.

Harley, G. (1989) Mind over body in cancer care. *Sunday Times*, 30 April.

Harner, M. (1988) What is a shaman? in *Shaman's Path: Healing, Personal Growth and Empowerment*, (ed. G. Doore), Shambhala, Boston, pp. 7–15.

Harner, M. (1988) Shamanic counselling, in *Shaman's Path: Healing Personal Growth and Empowerment*, (ed. G. Doore), Shambhala, Boston, pp. 179–88.

Harner, M. (1990) *The Way of the Shaman: A Guide to Power and Healing*. Harper & Row, New York.

Harris, G.W. (1955) *Neural Control of the Pituitary Gland*. Arnold, London.

Hartman, F. (1973) *Paracelsus: Life and Prophecies*. Rudog, Blauveit, New York.

Harwood, R. (1984) *All the World's a Stage*. Secker and Warburg, London.

Hawking, S.W. (1988) *A Brief History of Time: from the Big Bang to Black Holes*. Bantam, London.

Hay, L.L. (1988) *You Can Heal Your Life*. Eden Grove, London.

Hearnshaw, L.S. (1989) *The Shaping of Modern Psychology: An Historical Introduction*. Routledge, London.

Heil, M., Rosler F. and Hennghausen, E. (1993) Imagery–perception interaction depends on the shape of the image: a reply to Farah (1989). *J. Exp. Psychol. Human Perception and Performance*, **19** (6), 1313–20.

Hemery, D. (1978) Interviewed by Sir John Whitmore. *New Life Magazine*, Autumn, 21–5.

Hengartner, M.D. (1992) *Caenorhabditis elegans* gene ced-9. *Nature*, **356**, 494–9.

Herberman, R.B. (1982) Possible effects of central nervous system on natural killer (NK) cell activity, in *Biological Mediators of Behavior and Disease Neoplasia*, (ed. S.M. Levy), Elsevier, New York.

Herberman, R.B. *et al.* (1982) Interferons and NK cells, in *Interferons*, (eds T.C. Merigan and R.M. Friedman), Academic Press, London.

Herzfeld, G.M. and Taub, E. (1980) Effect of slide projections and tape-recorded suggestions on thermal biofeedback training. *Biofeedback and Individual Differences*, **1**, 129–33.

Heutzer, C.S. (1984) The power of meaning: from quantum mechanics to synchronicity. *J. Humanistic Psychology*, **24**, 80–94.

Hilgard, E.R. and Hilgard, J.R. (1975) *Hypnosis in the Relief of Pain*. W. Kaufman, Los Altos, California.

Hilgard, J.R. and le Baron, S. (1984) *Hypnotherapy of Pain in Children With Cancer*. W. Kaufman, Los Altos, California.

Hillman, J. (1975) *Re-visioning Psychology*. Harper Colophon, New York.

Hirai, T. (1975) *Zen Meditation Therapy*. Japan Publications, Tokyo.

Hirschman, R. and Favaro, L. (1986) Individual differences in imagery vividness and voluntary heart rate control. *Personality and Individual Differences*, **1**, 129–33.

Hnatiow, M. and Lang, P.J. (1965) Learned stabilization of heart rate. *Psychophysiology*, **1**, 330–6.

Hochheimer, W. (1969) *The Psychotherapy of C.G. Jung*. Translated by Hildegard Nagel, G.P. Putnam, New York, for the C.G. Jung Foundation for Analytical Psychology.

Hogan, R. and Kirchner, J. (1967) Preliminary report on the extinction of learned fears via short-term implosive therapy. *J. Abnormal Psychology*, **72**, 106–9.

Holden, C. (1981) Human-animal relationship under scrutiny. *Science*, **214**, 418–20.

Holden, R. (1992) Laughter: the best medicine? Presentation to the Second Annual Conference for the Promotion of Mental Health, Keele University.

Holt, R.R. (1964) Imagery: the return of the ostracized. *Am. Psychologist*, **12**, 254–64.

Holton, G. (1972) On trying to understand scientific genius. *Am. Scholar*, **41**, 95–110.

Honsberger, E. and Wilson, A.F. (1973) Transcendental Meditation in treating asthma: Respiration therapy. *J. Inhalation Technology*, **3**, 79–81.

Horn, S. (1986) *Relaxation: Modern Techniques for Stress Management.* Thorsons, Wellingborough, Northants.

Horowitz, M.I. (1970) *Image Formation and Cognition.* Butterworths, London.

Horowitz, M.J. (1978) Control of visual imagery and therapeutic intervention, in *The Power of the Imagination*, (eds J.L. Singer and K.S. Pope), Plenum, New York.

Houston, J. (1982) *The Possible Human.* J.P. Tarcher, Los Angeles.

Hucklebridge, F.H. (1990) Simulation of human peripeheral lymphocytes by methionine-enkephaline and E-selective opioid analogues. *Immunopharmacology*, **19**, 87–91.

Hucklebridge, F. (1993) Psychoneuroimmunology. Presentation to Biology Department, Keele University, 3 February.

Hudson, L. (1972) *The Cult of the Fact.* Cape, London.

Hughes, J. (1987) *Cancer and Emotion: Psychological Preludes and Reactions to Cancer.* Wiley, Chichester.

Humphrey, M.E. and Zangwill, O.L. (1951) Cessation of dreaming after brain injury. *J. Neurology, Neurosurgery and Psychiatry*, **14**, 322–5.

Humphreys, C. (1962) *Zen.* Hodder & Stoughton, London.

Hunt, I. and Draper, W.W. (1964) *Lightning In His Hand: the life story of Nicola Tesla.* Sage Books, Denver, Colorado.

Hunter, I.M.L. (1986) Exceptional memory skill, in *The Skilful Mind*, (ed. A. Gellatly), Open University Press, Milton Keynes, pp. 76–86.

Huxley, A. (1954) *The Doors of Perception.* Chatto & Windus, London.

Huxley, A. (1977) Moksha: writings on psychedelics and visionary experience (1931–1963). Stonehill Publishing, New York.

Ikeda, Y. and Hirai, H. (1976) Voluntary control of electrodermal activity in relation to imagery and internal perception scores. *Psychophysiology*, **13**, 330–3.

Illich, I. (1975) *Medical Nemesis: the Expropriation of Health.* Marion Boyars, London.

Inglis, B. (1987) *The Unknown Guest.* Chatto & Windus, London.

Inglis, B. (1990) *Trance: a Natural History of Altered States of Mind.* Paladin, London.

Jackson, D. (1993) You'd better believe in the bogeyman. *Independent*, 3 March.

Jackson, R. (1992) Psychotherapy: beyond a phoney love. *Leading Edge*, **6**, 14–15.

Jacobi, J. (1962) *The Psychology of Jung.* Routledge and Kegan Paul, London.

Jacobs, M. (1992) *Sigmund Freud.* Sage, London.

Jacobs, T.J. and Charles, E. (1980) Life events and the occurrence of cancer in children. *Psychosomatic Med.*, **42**, 1–24.

Jacobsen, C.F. (1936) Studies of cerebral function in primates 1: The functions of the frontal association areas in monkeys. *Comp. Psychol. Monogr.*, **13**, 3–60.

Jacobsen, E. (1929) Electrical measurements of neuromuscular states during mental activities: imagination of movement involving skeletal muscle. *Am. J. Physiology*, **91**, 597–608.

Jacq, C. (1985) *Egyptian Magic.* Avis and Phillips, Warminster.

Jaffe, D.T. and Bresler, D.E. (1980) Guided imagery: healing through the mind's eye, in *Imagery: Its Many Dimensions and Applications*, (eds J.E. Shorr, G.E. Sobel, P. Robin and J.A. Connella), Plenum, New York.

Jamal, M. (1987) *Shape Shifters*. Arkana, London.

Jaynes, J. (1993) *The Origin of Consciousness in the Breakdown of the Bicameral Mind*. Penguin, Harmondsworth.

Jemmott, J.B. *et al.* (1983) Academic stress, power motivation and decrease in salivary immunoglobin A secretion rate. *Lancet*, **1**, 1400–2.

Jemmott, J.B. and Locke, S.E. (1984) Psychosocial factors, immunologic mediation and human susceptibility to infectious disease: How much do we know? *Psychological Bull.*, **95**, 78–108.

Jensen, M.M. and Rasmussen, A.F. (Jr) (1963) Stress and susceptibility to viral infections II: Sound stress and susceptibility to vesicular stomatatis virus. *J. Immunology*, **90**, 21–3.

Joasoo, A. and McKenzie, J.M. (1976) Stress and the immune response in rats. *Int. Arch. Allergy Appl. Immunol.*, **50**, 659–663.

Johnson, H,E. and Gorton, W.H. (1973) A practical method of muscle reeducation in hemiphlegia: electromyographic facilitation. Unpublished manuscript. Casa Colina Hospital for Rehabilitation Medicine, Paloma, California, cited in Pelletier (1978).

Jones, G.E. and Johnson, H.J. (1978) Physiological responding during self-generated imagery of contextually complete stimuli. *Psychophysiology*, **15**, 439–46.

Jones, G.E. and Johnston, H.J. (1980) Heart rate and somatic concomitants of mental imagery. *Psychophysiology*, **17**, 339–47.

Jordan, C.S. and Lenington, K.T. (1979) Physiological correlates of eidetic imagery and induced anxiety. *J. Mental Imagery*, **3**, 31–42.

Jourard, S. (1971) *The Transparent Self*. Van Nostrand, New York.

Jung, C.G. (1946) *Psychology and Religion*. Yale University Press, New Haven.

Jung, C,G. (1954) *The Archetypes and the Collective Unconscious. The Collected Works of C.G. Jung, Vol. 9*. Princeton University Press, Princeton, New Jersey.

Jung, C.G. (1955) *Mysterium Coniunctionis. Vol 14. Collected works*. Princeton University Press, Princeton, New Jersey.

Jung, C.G. (1959) Face to Face with C.G. Jung. BBC Interview first broadcast October 1959, repeated 16 October 1988.

Jung, C.G. (1960) *The Structure and Dynamics of the Unconscious. Collected Works Vol.8*. Princeton University Press, Princeton, New Jersey.

Jung, C.G. (1963) *The Integration of the Personality*. 9th impression. Translated by S.Dell. Routledge and Kegan Paul, London.

Jung, C.G. (1966) *Modern Man in Search of a Soul*. Routledge and Kegan Paul, London.

Jung, C.G. (1967) *Symbols of Transformation. Collected works, Vol. 2*. 2nd edn. Princeton University Press, Princeton, New Jersey.

Jung, C.G. (1971) *The Archetypes and the Collective Unconscious*. Translated by R.F.C. Hull. Routledge, London.

Jung, C.G. (1972a) *Memories, Dreams, Reflections*. Translated by R. and C. Winston. Collins, Fontana, Glasgow.

Jung, C.G. (1972b) *Synchronicity: An acausal connecting principle*. Translated by R.F.C. Hull. Routledge and Kegan Paul, London.

Jung, C.G. (1976) *The Symbolic Life*. Princeton University Press, Princeton, New Jersey.

Jung, C.G. (1978) *Psychology and the East*. Routledge and Kegan Paul, London.

Kakar, S. (1984) *Shamans, Mystics and Doctors: a Psychological Enquiry into India and its Healing Traditions*. George Allen and Unwin, London.

Kalweit, H. (1988) *Dreamtime and Inner Space: the World of the Shaman*. Translated by W. Wunsche. Shambhala, Boston.

Kamiya, J. (1968) Consicous control of brain waves. *Psychology Today*, **1**, 57–60.

Kamiya, J. (1969) Operant control of the EEG alpha rhythm and some of its reported effects on consciousnessness, in *Altered States of Consciousness*. (ed. C.T. Tart), Wiley, New York.

Kaptehuk, T. and Croucher, M. (1986) *The Healing Arts: a Journey Through the Faces of Medicine*. BBC Publications, London.

Karamatsu, A. and Hirai, T. (1966) Studies of EEGS of expert zen meditators. *Folia Psychiatrica Neurologica Japonica*, **28**, 315.

Karamatsu, A. and Hirai, T. (1969) An electroencephalographic study of zen meditation (zazen), in *Altered States of Consciousness*, (ed. C. Tart), Wiley, New York, pp. 489–502.

Kasl, S.V., Evans, A.S. and Neiderman, J.C. (1979) Psychological risk factors in the development of infectious mononucleosis. *Psychosomatic Med.*, **41**, 445–66.

Kazdin, A.E. and Wilcoxin, L.A. (1975) Systematic desensitization and non-sepcific treatment effects: a methodological evaluation. *Psychological Bull.*, **83**, 5.

Kelley, H.H. (1950) The warm-cold variable in first impressions of people. *J. Personality*, **18**, 431–9.

Kelly, C.R. (1961) Psychological factors in myopia. Proceedings of the American Psychological Association, 31 August.

Kennedy, S., Kiecolt-Glaser, J.K. and Glaser, R. (1988) Immunological consequences of acute and chronic stressors: mediating role of interpersonal relationships. *Br. J. Med. Psychology*, **61**, 77–85.

Kent, G. (1986) Hypnosis in dentistry. *Br. J. Exp. Clin. Hypnosis*, **3**, 103–12.

Kepecs, J.G. (1954) Observations on screens and barriers in the mind. *Psychoanalytic Quarterly*, **23**, 62–77.

Kerr, J.F.R., Wylie, A. and Currie, A. (1972) Apoptosis: A basic biological phenomenon. *Br. J. Cancer*, **26**, 239–57.

Kiecolt-Glaser, J. *et al.* (1984) Psychosocial modifiers of immunocompetence in medical students. *Psychosomatic Med.*, **46** (1), 7–14.

Kiecolt-Glaser, J.K., *et al.* (1986) Modulation of cellular immunity in medical students. *J. Behavioural Med.*, **9**, 5–21.

Kiecolt-Glaser, J.K. *et al.* (1985) Psychosocial enhancement of immunoincompetence in a geriatric population. *Health Psychology*, **4**, 25–41.

Kiesler, E. (1984) The playing fields of the mind. *Psychology Today*, 18 July, 18–24.

King, S. (1983) *Kahuna Healing*. Theosophical Publishing House, Wheaton, Illinois.

Kissen, D.M. and Eysenck, H.J. (1962) Personality in male lung cancer patients. *Br. J. Med. Psychology*, **36**, 123–7.

Kissen, D.M. and Eysenck, H.J. (1963) Personal characteristics in males conducive to lung cancer. *Br. J. Med. Psychology*, **36**, 27–36.

Kissen, D.M. and Eysenck, H.J. (1964) Relationship between lung cancer, cigarette smoking, inhalation and personality. *Br. J. Med. Psychology*, **27**, 203–16.

Kissen, D.M. and Eysenck, H.J. (1967) Psychosocial factors, personality and lung cancer in men aged 55–64. *Br. J. Med. Psychology*, **40**, 26–43.

Kleiger, J.H. and Kinsman, R.A. (1980) The development of the MMPI alexithymia scale. *Psychotherapy and Psychosomatics*, **34** (1), 17–24.

Klinger, E. (1971) *The Structure and Function of Fantasy*. Wiley, New York.

Koestler, A. (1976) *The Call Girls: a Tragi-comedy with Prologue and Epilogue*. Pan Books, London.

Koestler, A. (1984) *The Sleepwalkers: a history of man's changing vision of the universe*. Penguin, Harmondsworth.

Kolvin, I. (1967) Aversive imagery treatment in adolescents. *Behavioural Res. Therapy*, **5**, 245–8.

Kosslyn, S.M. (1980) *Image and Mind*. Harvard University Press, Cambridge, Massachussetts.

Kosslyn, S.M. *et al.* (1985) A computational analysis of mental image generation: evidence from functional dissociations in split brain patients. *J. Exp. Psychology: General*, **114**, 311–41.

Kretschmer, W. (1969) Meditative techniques in psychotherapy, in *Altered States of Consciousness: a Book of Readings*, (ed. C. Tart), Wiley, New York, pp. 219–31.

Krippner, S. (1988) The first healers, in *Shaman's Path: Healing, Personal Growth and Empowerment*, (ed. G. Doore), Shambhala, London, pp. 101–14.

Krystal, P. (1982) *Cutting The Ties That Bind: How to Achieve Liberation from False Security and Negative Conditioning*. Element, Shaftesbury, Dorset.

Krystal, P. (1990) *Cutting More Ties That Bind: Educating Children and Reprogramming Adults*. Element, Shaftesbury, Dorset.

Kubler-Ross, E. (1982) *Working It Through*. MacMillan, New York.

Kunzendorf, R.G. (1981) Individual differences in imagery and autonomic control. *J. Mental Imagery*, **5**, 47–60.

Kunzendorf, R.G. and Bradbury, J.L. (1983) Better liars have better imaginations. *Psychological Rep.*, **52**, 634.

Kunzendorf, R.G. (1984) Centrifugal effects of eidetic imaging on flash electroretinograms and autonomic responses. *J. Mental Imagery*, **8**, 67–76.

Laing, R.D. (1959) *The Divided Self: An Existential Study of Sanity and Madness*. Tavistock, London.

Laing, R.D. (1983) *The Voice of Experience: Experience, Science and Psychiatry*. Allen Lane, London.

Laing, R.D. (1991) Did you used to be R.D. Laing? Channel 4. 27 April.

Lang, P.J. (1967) Effects of feedback and instructional set. *J. Exp. Psychology*, **75**, 425.

Lang, P.J. *et al.* (1980) Emotional imagery: conceptual structure and pattern of somatovisceral response. *Psychophysiology*, **17**, 179–92.

Laws, D.R. and Rubin, H.B. (1969) Instructional control of an autonomic sexual response. *J. Appl. Behav.-Analysis*, **2**, 93–9.

Lazarus, R.S. (1966) *Psychological Stress and the Coping Process*. McGraw Hill, New York.

LeBouef, A. and Wilson, C. (1978) The importance of imagery in maintenance of feedback-assisted relaxation over extinction trials. *Perceptual Motor Skills*, **47**, 824–6.

Le Carré, J. (1989) *The Russia House*. Hodder & Stoughton, London.

LeShan, L. (1959) Psychological states as factors in the development of malignant disease: a critical review. *J. Natl. Cancer Inst.*, **22**, 1–18.

LeShan, L. (1966) An emotional life-history pattern associated with neoplastic disease. *Ann. New York Acad. Sci.*, **125**, 780–93.

LeShan, L. (1969) Physicists and mystics: similarities in world view. *J. Transpersonal Psychology*, **1** (2), 1–20.

LeShan, L. (1974) *The Medium, the Mystic and the Physicist: Towards a General Theory of the Paranormal*. Viking Press, New York.

LeShan, L. (1982) *Clairvoyant Reality: towards a general theory of the paranormal*. Turnstone Press, Wellingborough, Northants.

Leuner, H. (1977) Guided affective imagery: an account of its development. *J. Mental Imagery*, **1**, 73–92.

Leuner, H. (1978) Basic principles an therapeutic efficacy of Guided Affective Imagery, in *The Power of the Human Imagination*, (eds J.L. Singer and K.S. Pope), Plenum, New York.

Leuner, H. (1984) *Guided Affective Imagery*. Thieme-Stratton, New York.

LeVine, D.N., Warach, J. and Farah, M.J. (1985) Two visual systems in mental imagery: Dissociation of 'what' and 'where' in imagery disorders due to bilateral posterior cerebral lesions. *Neurology*, **35**, 1010–8.

Lévy-Bruhl, L. (1928) *The 'Soul' of the Primitive*. Allen and Unwin, London.

Lewis, J.H. and Sarbin, T.R. (1943) Studies in psychosomatics. *Psychosomatic Med.*, **5**, 125.

Ley, R.G. (1983) Cerebral laterality and imagery, in *Imagery, Current Theory, Research and Application*, (ed. A.A. Sheikh), Wiley, New York.

Ley, R.G. and Bryden, M.P. (1983) Right hemispheric involvement in imagery and affect, in *Cognitive Processing in the Right Hemisphere*, (ed. E. Perecman), Academic Press, New York.

Ley, R.G. and Smylie, M. (1989) Cerebral laterality: implications for Eastern and Western therapies, in *Eastern and Western Approaches to Healing: Ancient Wisdom and Modern Knowledge*, (eds A.A. Sheikh and K.S. Sheikh), Wiley, New York, pp. 325–43.

Lilly, J.C. (1973) *The Centre of the Cyclone: an Autobiography of Inner Space*. Paladin, London.

Lilly, J.C. (1977) *The Deep Self*. Simon and Schuster, New York.

Linden, W. (1973) Practising of meditation by school children and their levels of field dependence – independence, test anxiety and reading achievement. *J. Consulting Clin. Psychology*, **41**, 139–43.

Lovelock, J.E. (1979) *Gaia*. Oxford University Press, London.

Lucas, O. (1965) Dental extractions in the hemophiliac: control of the emotional factors by hypnosis. *Am. J. Clin. Hypnosis*, **7**, 301–7.

Luthe, W. (1969) Autogenic Training, method, research and application in medicine, in *Altered States of Consciousness: a Book of Readings*, (ed. C. Tart), Wiley, New York, pp. 309–19,

Lyles, J. *et al.* (1982) Efficacy of relaxation training and guided imagery in reducing the aversiveness of cancer chemotherapy. *J. Consulting Clin. Psychology*, **50** (4), 509–24.

Macbeth, J. (1991) *Sun Over Mountain: a Course in Creative Imagination*. Gateway Books, Bath.

McCanne, T.R. and Iennarella, R.S. (1980) Cognitive and somatic events associated with discriminative changes in heart rate. *Psychophysiology*, **17**, 18–28.

McClelland, D.C. *et al.* (1982) The need for power, stress, immune function and illness among male prisoners. *J. Abnormal Psychology*, **91**, 61–70.

McClelland, D.C. and Jemmott, J.B. (1980) Power motivation stress and physical illness. *J. Human Stress*, **6**, 6–15.

McClelland, D.C. *et al.* (1980) Stressed power motivation, sympathetic activation, immune function and illness. *J. Human Stress*, **6**, 11–19.

McClelland, D.C. and Kirshcnit, C. (1984) The effect of motivational arousal through films on salivary immune function. Unpublished paper, Harvard University Department of Psychology and Social Relations, Cambridge, MA, cited in Pelletier and Herzing 1989.

McCulloch, M.I. (1982) Animal facilitated therapy: an overview. *California Veterinarian*, **8**, 13–24.

McKellar, P. (1968) *Experience and Behaviour*. Penguin, Harmondsworth.

McKellar, P. (1989) Abnormal Psychology: its experience and behaviour. Seminar, Psychology Department, Keele University, 8 May.

McMahon, C.E. and Sheikh, A.A. (1984) Imagination in disease and healing processes: a historical perspective, in *Imagination and Healing*, (ed. A.A. Sheikh), Baywood, Farmingdale, New York.

Mangan, G.L. (1974) Personality and conditioning: some personality, cognitive and psychophysiological parameters of classical (appetitive) sexual GSR conditioning. *Pavlovian J. Biol. Sci.*, **9**, 125–35.

Manning, M. (1988) Seminar on self-healing. Presented at Holistic Health Workshop, Farnham Holistic Health Centre, 30 April.

Manning, M. (1989) *Matthew Manning's Guide to Self-healing*. Thorsons, Wellinborough, Northants.

Marchand, H. (1956) Die suggestion der warme im oberbauch und ihr einfluss auf blutzucker und leukozytem. *Psychotherapie*, **3**, 154.

Marchand, H. (1961) Das verhalten von blutzucker und leukozyten wahrend des autogenen trainings, in Proceedings of the Third International Congress of Psychiatry, Montreal.

Marinacci, A.A. (1968) *Applied Electromyography*. Lea and Febiger, Philadelphia.

Marks, I. and Gelder, M.G. (1967) Transvestitism and fetishism: clinical and psychological changes during faradic aversion. *Br. J. Psychiatry*, **113**, 711–29.

Marks, I. *et al.* (1971) Physiological accompaniments of mental and phobic imagery. *Psychological Med.*, **1**, 299–307.

Marks, I. and Huson, J. (1973) Physiological aspects of neutral and phobic imagery: Further observations. *Br. J. Psychiatry*, **122**, 567–72.

Marzillier, J.S., Carroll, D. and Newland, J.R. (1979) Self-report and physiological changes accompanying repeated imaging of a phobic scene. *Behaviour Res. Therapy*, **17**, 71–7.

Maslow, A.H. (1968) *Towards a Psychology of Being*. Van Nostrand, New York.

Mauz, F. (1948) The psychotic man. *Arch. psychiatrie*.

Meares, A. (1977) Atavistic regression as a factor in the remision of cancer. *Med. J. Australia*, **2**, 32–133.

Meares, A. (1981) Regression or recurrence of carcinoma of the breast at mastectomy site associated with intensive meditation. *Australian Family Physician*, **10**, 2181–9.

Meichenbaum, D. (1978) Why does using imagery in psychotherapy lead to change? in *The Power of Human Imagination*. (eds J.L. Singer and K.S. Pope), Plenum, New York.

Medik, L. and Fursland, A. (1984) Maximising scarce resources: autogenic relaxation classes at a health centre. *Br. J. Med. Psychology*, **57**, 181–5.

Menzies, R. (1937) Conditioned vasomotor responses in human subjects. *J. Exp. Psychology*, **4**, 75–120.

Menzies, R. (1941) Further studies of conditioned vasomotor responses in human subjects. *J. Exp. Psychology*, **29**, 457–82.

Metzler, J. and Shepard, R.N. (1974) Transformational studies of the internal representation of 3-dimensional objects, in *Theories in Cognitive Psychology: The Loyola Symposium*, (ed. R. Solos), Erlbaum, Potomac, Maryland.

Meyer, A. and Beck, F. (1954) *Prefrontal Leucotomy and Relation Operations: Anatomic Aspects of Success or Failure*. Chas. C. Thomas, Springfiled, Illinois.

Miller, M.V. (1989) Introduction to 'Gestalt Therapy Verbatim'. *Gestalt J.*, **12** (1), 5–24.

Miller, N.E. (1969) Learning of visceral and glandular responses. *Science*, **163**, 434–45.

Millson, P. and Malone, D. (eds) (1994) *Death Wish – The Untold Story*. Broadcasting Support Services, London.

Milner, B. (1971) Interhemispheric differences in the localization of psychological processes. *Br. Med. Bull.*, **27**, 272–7.

Mohamed, M.A. and Hanson, R.P. (1980) Effect of social stress on Newcastle disease virus (La Sota) infection. *Avian Disease*, **24**, 908–15.

Money, M. (1992) The shamanic path to mental health. Paper presented at The Second Annual Conference for the Promotion of Mental Health, Keele University, September.

Monjo, de, V.P. (1987) The conditions of yoga therapy, in *The Art of Survival: A Guide to Yoga Therapy*, (eds. D. Gharote and M. Lockart), Unwin Hyman, London, pp. 66–78.

Moon, T. and Moon, H. (1984) Hypnosis and childbirth: self-report and comment. *Br. J. Exp. Clin. Hypnosis*, **1**, 49–52.

Moos, R.H. (1964a) Personality factors associated with rheumatoid arthritis: review. *J. Chronic Disorders*, **17**, 41.

Moos, R.H. and Solomon, G.F. (1964b) Personality correlates of the rapidity of progression of rheumatoid arthritis. *Ann. Rheumatic Disease*, **23**, 145–51.

Moos, R.H. and Solomon, G.F. (1964c) Minnestota Multiphasic Personality Inventory response patterns in patients with Rheumatoid Arthritis. *J. Psychosomatic Res.*, **8**, 145–151.

Moos, R.H. and Solomon, G.F. (1965a) Psychological comparisons between women with rheumatoid arthritis and their non-arthritic sisters I: Personality and interview rating data. *Psychosomatic Med.*, **27**, 135.

Moos, R.H. and Solomon, G.F. (1965b) Psychological comparisons between women with rheumatoid arthritis and their non-arthritic sisters II: Content analysis of interviews. *Psychosomatic Med.*, **27**, 150.

Morgan, G. (1993) *Imaginization: The Art of Creative Management*. Sage, London.

Motoyama, M. (1987) Yoga and acupuncture, in *A Guide to Yoga Therapy*, (eds. M.I. Gharote and M. Lockart), Unwin Hyman, London, pp. 107–15.

Mugford, R.A. and McComisky, J.G. (1975) Some recent work on the psychotherautic value of caged bird with old people, in *Pet Animals and Society*, (ed. R.S. Andersen), Bailliere Tindall, London.

Muller-Hegemann, D. and Kohler, C. (1961) Eight years experience with Autogenic Training, in Proceedings of The Third International Congress of Psychiatry, Montreal.

Muslin, H.L., Gyarfas, K. and Pieper, W.J. (1966) Separation experience and cancer of the breast. *Ann. New York Acad. Sci.*, **125**, 802–6.

Naish, P.L. (1986) *What is Hypnosis? Current Theories and Research.* Open University Press, Milton Keynes.

Nevis, E. (1992) *Organizational Consulting: A Gestalt Approach.* Gardner Press, New York.

Nidich, S., Seeman, W. and Dreskin, T. (1973) Influence of transcendental meditation: A replication. *J. Counselling Psychology*, **20**, 565–6.

Norris, P. (1989) Current conceptual trends in biofeedback and self-regulation, in *Eastern and Western Approaches to Healing Ancient Wisdom and Modern Knowledge*, (eds A.A. Sheikh and K.S. Sheikh), Wiley, New York, pp. 264–95.

Nunn, T.H. (1822) *Cancer of the Breast.* J. & A. Churchill, London.

Oaklander, V. (1978) *Windows to Our Children: A Gestalt Therapy Approach to Children and Adolescents.* Real People's Press, Utah.

Ogden, J.A. (1985) Contralesional neglect of constructed visual images in right and left brain-damaged patients. *Neuropsychologia*, **23**, 273–7.

Okhuma, Y. (1985) Effects of evoking imagery on the control of peripheral skin temperature. *Japanese J. Psychology*, **54**, 88–94 (English abstract).

Oldham, J. (1989) Psychological support for cancer patients. *Br. J. Occupational Ther.*, **52** (12), 463–65.

Orme-Johnson, D.W. (1973) Autonomic ability and Transcendental Meditation. *Psychosomatic Med.*, **35**, 341–9.

Orne, M.T. (1959) The nature of hypnosis: artifact and essence. *J. Abnormal Social Psychology*, **58**, 277–99.

Ornstein, R.E. (1972) *The Psychology of Consciousness.* Freeman, San Francisco, California.

Ornstein, R.E. *et al.* (1979) Differential right hemisphere involvement in two reading tasks. *Psychophysiology*, **16**, 398–401.

Ornstein, R.E. and Sobel, D. (1988) *The Healing Brain: A Radical New Approach to Health Care.* MacMillan, London.

Pagels, H.R. (1983) *The Cosmic Code: Quantum Physics as the Language of Nature.* Michael Joseph, London.

Paget, J. (1870) *Surgical Pathology.* 2nd edn., Longman, Brown Green and Longman, London.

Paiva, T. *et al.* (1982) Effects of frontalis EMG biofeedback and Diazepam in the treatment of tension headache. *Headache*, **22**, 216–20.

Paivio, A. (1971) *Imagery and Verbal Processes.* Holt, Rinehart and Winston, New York.

Paivio, A. (1972) A theoretical analysis of the role of imagery in learning and memory, in *The Function and Nature of Imagery*, (ed. P.W. Sheehan), Academic Press, New York, pp. 253–75.

Paivio, A. (1989) A dual coding perspective on imagary and the brain, in *Neuropsychology of Visual Perception*, (ed. J.W. Brown), Lawrence Erlbaum and Associates, Hillsdale, New Jersey, pp. 203–16.

Palmblad, J. (1981) Stress and immunologic competence: studies in man, in *Psychoneuroimmunology*, (ed. R. Ader), Academic Press, New York, pp. 87–92.

Panagiotou, N. and Sheikh, A.A. (1977) The image and the unconscious. *Int. J. Social Psychiatry*, **23**, 169–86.

Parker, W. (1885) *Cancer: A study of cases of cancer of the female breast.* New York.

Passchier, J. and Helm-Hylkema, H. (1981) The effect of stress imagery on arousal and its implications for biofeedback of the frontalis muscles. *Biofeedback Self Regulation*, **6**, 295–303.

Patel, C.H. and Datey, K.K. (1975) Yoga and biofeedback in the management of hypertension: two control studies. Proceedings of the Biofeedback Res. Society, Monterey: California.

Patel, C.H. (1973) Yoga and biofeedback in the management of hypertension. *Lancet*, 10 November.

Paul, G. and Trimble, R. (1970) Recorded vs 'live' relaxation training and hypnotic suggestion: comparative effectiveness for reducing arousal and inhibiting stress responses. *Behaviour Therapy*, **1** (3), 285–302.

Peavey, B.S. (1982) Biofeedback assisted regulation: Effects on phagocytic immune functions. Unpublished doctoral thesis Texas State University, Denton, cited in Achterberg (1985).

Pelletier, K.R. and Herzing, D.L. (1989) Psychoneuroimmunology: Towards a mind-body model, in *Eastern and Western Approaches to Healing Ancient Wisdom and Modern Knowledge*, (eds A.A. Sheikh and K.S. Sheikh), Wiley, New York.

Pelletier, K.S. and Peper, E. (1977) Alpha EEG feedback as a means of pain control. *J. Clin. Exp. Hypnosis*, **25** (4), 361–71.

Pelletier, K.R. (1978) *Mind as Healer, Mind as Slayer: a Holistic Approach to Preventing Stress Disorders*. George, Allen and Unwin, London.

Perls, F.S. (1969) *Gestalt Therapy Verbatim*. Bantam, New York.

Perls, F.S. (1973) *Gestalt Therapy*. Penguin, Harmondsworth.

Perls, F.S. (1976) *The Gestalt Approach and Eye Witness to Therapy*. Bantam, New York.

Pert, C.B. (1986) The wisdom of the receptors: neuropeptides, the emotions and body-mind. *Advances*, **3** (3), 8–16.

Pert, C.B. (1987) Neuropeptides: the emotions and bodymind, *Noetic Sci Rev.*, **2**, 13–18.

Peters, F. (1964) *Boyhood With Gurdjieff*. Dutton, London.

Peters, F. (1965) *Gurdjieff Remembered*. Gollancz, London.

Peters, F. (1978) *Balanced Man: A Look at Gurdjieff Fifty Years Later*. Wildwood, London.

Peters, L.G. and Price-Williams. D. (1980) Towards an experiential analysis of shamanism. *Am. Ethnologist*, **7**, 398–418.

Pickett, E. (1987–1988) Fibroid tumors: a response to guided imagery and music: two case studies. *Imagination, Cognition Personality*, **7**, 165–76.

Pilisik, M. and Parks, S.H. (1986) *The Healing Web: Social Networks and Human Survival*. University Press of New England.

Pirsig, R.M. (1974) *Zen and the Art of Motorcycle Maintenance*. The Bodley Head, London.

Polanyi, M. (1958) *Personal Knowledge: Towards a Post-critical Philosophy*. Routledge and Kegan Paul, London.

Polzein, P. (1961a) Electrocardiographic changes during the first standard exercise, in Proceedings of the Third Congress of Psychiatry, Montreal.

Polzien, P. (1961b) Respiratory changes during passive concentraton on heaviness, in Proceedings of the Third Congress of Psychiatry, Montreal.

Polzein, P. (1961c) Therapeutic possibilities of Autogenic Training in hyperthyroid conditions, in Proceedings of the Third Congress of Psychiatry, Montreal.

Prabhupado, Swami, (1968) *Bhagavad Gita As It Is*. The Bhaktivedanta Book Trust, New York.

Pribram, K.H. (1978) *Languages of the Brain: Experimental Paradoxes and Principles in Neuropsychology*. Prentice Hall, Englewood Cliffs, New Jersey.

Priestman, T.J., Priestman, S.G. and Bradshaw, C. (1985) Stress and breast cancer. *Br. J. Cancer*, **51**, 493–8.

Progoff, I. (1963) *The Symbolic and the Real*. Julian Press, New York.

Progoff, I. (1970) Waking dream and living myth, in *Myths, Dreams and Religion*, (ed. J. Campbell), Dutton, New York.

Prosser, G.V., Carson, P. and Phillips, R. (1985) Exercise after myocardial infarction: Long-term rehabilitation effects. *J. Psychosomatic Res.*, **29** (5), 535–40.

Pylyshyn, Z. (1973) What the mind's eye tells the mind's brain: a critique of mental imagery. *Psychological Bull.*, **80**, 1–24.

Pylyshyn, Z. (1981) The imagery debate:analogue media versus tacit knowledge. *Psychological Rev.*, **87**, 16–45.

Qualls, P.J. and Sheehan, P.W. (1979) Capacity for absorption and relaxation during electromyograph biofeedback and no feedback conditions. *J. Abnormal Psychology*, **88**, 652–62.

Qualls, P.J. and Sheehan, P.W. (1981a) Imagery encouragement, absorption capacity and relaxation during electromyograph biofeedback. *J. Personality Social Psychology*, **41**, 370–9.

Qualls, P.J. and Sheehan, P.W. (1981b) Role of feedback signal in electromyograph feedback: the relevance of attention. *J. Exp. Psychology: General*, **110**, 204–16.

Raff, M.C. (1992) Social controls on cell survival and cell death. *Nature*, **356**, 397–400.

Rajneesh, Bhagwan Shree (1979) *Take It Easy Vol. I. Talks of Zen Buddhism*. Rajneesh Foundation, Poona.

Redd, W.H., Andersen, G.V. and Minagawa, R.Y. (1982) Hypnotic control of anticipatory emesis in patients receiving cancer chemotherapy. *J. Consulting Clin. Psychology*, **50** (1), 14–19.

Reich, W. (1975) *Reich Speaks of Freud*. Penguin, Harmondsworth.

Reid, D. (1985) Japanese religions, in *A Handbook of Living Religions*, (ed. J.H. Hinnells), Penguin, Harmondsworth, pp. 344–64.

Reite, M., Harbeck, R. and Hoffman, A. (1981) Altered cellular immune response following peer separation. *Life Sci*, **29**, 1133–6.

Renneker, R.E. *et al.* (1963) Psychoanalytic explorations of emotional correlates of cancer of the breast. *Psychosomatic Med.*, **25**, 96–108.

Revland, P. and Hirschman, R. (1976) Imagery training and visual biofeedback. *Psychophysiology*, **13**, 186–7.

Reyher, J. (1963) Free imagery, an uncovering procedure. *J. Clin. Psychology*, **19**, 454–9.

Reyher, J. (1977) Spontaneous visual imagery: implications for psychoanalysis, psychopathology and psychotherapy. *J. Mental Imagery*, **2**, 253–74.

Rider, M.S., Floyd, J.W. and Kirkpatrick, J. (1985) The effect of music, imagery and relaxation as on adrenal corticosteroids and the retentrainment of circadian rhythms. *J. Music Therapy*, **22**, 46–58.

Riley, V. (1981) Psychoneuroendocrine influences on immunocompetence and neoplasia. *Science*, **212**, 1100–9.

Roberts, A.H., Kewman, D.G. and MacDonald, H. (1973) Voluntary control of skin temperatures: unilateral changes using hypnosis and feedback. *J. Abnormal Psychology*, **82**, 163–8.

Roberts, R.J. and Weerts, T.C. (1982) Cardiovascular responding during anger and fear imagery. *Psychological Reports*, **50**, 219–30.

Roet, B. (1987) *All In The Mind*. MacDonald, Optima, London.

Roet, B. (1988) Address given at the World Health Day, Holistic Health Centre, Farnham, England.

Roos, P.E. and Cohen, L.H. (1987) Sex roles and social support as moderators of life stress adjustment. *J. Personality Social Psychology*, **52**, 576–85.

Rosch, P.J. (1984) Stress and cancer, in *Psychosocial Stress and Cancer*, (ed. C.L. Cooper), Wiley, Chichester.

Rose, S., Kamin, L.J. and Lewontin, R.C. (1984) *Not In Our Genes: Biology, Ideology and Human Nature*. Penguin, Harmondsworth.

Rossi, E.L. (1986) *The Psychobiology of Mind-Body Healing: New Concepts in Therapeutic Hypnosis*. W.W. Norton, New York.

Roszak, T. (1970) *The Making of a Counter Culture: Reflections on the Culture and its Youthful Opposition*. Faber and Faber, London.

Roszak, T. (1975) *Unfinished Animal: the Aquarian Frontier and the Evolution of Consciousness*. Harper & Row, New York.

Roth, G. (1990–1991) An urban shaman. *Kindred Spirit*, **2** (1), 33–7.

Russell, B. (1948) *History of Western Philosophy and its Connection with Political and Social Circumstances from the Earliest Times to the Present Day*. Allen and Unwin, London.

Russell, B. (1959) *Mysticism and Logic and Other Essays*. Allen and Unwin, London.

Sacerdote, P. (1982) Techniques of hypnotic intervention with pain patients. *Ann. New York Acad. Sci.*, **125** (3), 101–19.

Sarason, I.G., Sarason, B.R. and Pierce, G.R. (1988) Social support, personality and health, in *Topics in Health Psychology*, (eds S. Maes, C.D. Spielberger, P.B. Defares and I.G. Sarason), Wiley, New York, pp. 245–55.

Sarason, B.R., Sarason, I.G. and Pierce, G.R. (1990) *Social Support: A Transactional View*. Wiley, New York.

Sarbin, T.R. (1962) Attempts to understand hypnotic phenomena, in *Psychology In The Making*, (ed. L. Postman), Knopf, New York, pp. 98–103.

Saso, M. (1985) Chinese religions, in *A Handbook of Living Religions*, (ed. J.H. Hinnells), Penguin, Harmondsworth, pp. 344–69.

Schleifer, S.J. *et al.* (1983) Suppression of lymphocyte stimulation following bereavement. *J. Am. Med. Assoc.*, **250**, 374–7.

Schleifer, S. *et al.* (1984) Lymphocyte function in major depressive disorders. *Arch. General Psychiatry*, **41**, 484–6.

Schmale, A. and Iker, S.H. (1966) The effect of hopelessness and the development of cancer. I. Identification of uterine cervical cancer in women with atypical cytology. *Psychosomatic Med.*, **28**, 714–21.

Schmale, R.B. and Iker, S.H. (1971) Hopelessness as a predictor of cervical cancer. *Social Sci. Med.*, **5**, 95–100.

Schneider, J. *et al.* (1988) Psychological factors influencing immune system function in normal subjects: A summary of research findings and implications for the use of guided imagery. Paper presented at the 10th Annual Conference of the Am. Association for the Study of Mental Imagery, New Haven, CT, cited in Sheikh, Kunzendorf and Sheikh (1989).

Schonfield, J. (1975) Psychology and life experience: differences between Israeli women with benign and cancerous breast lesions. *J. Psychosomatic Res.*, **19**, 229–34.

Schultz, J.H. (1932) *Das Autogene training.* Thieme Verlag, Stuttgart.

Schultz, J.H. and Luthe, W. (1959) *Autogenic Training: A Psychophysiological Approach to Psychotherapy.* Grune and Stratton, New York.

Schultz, J.H. and Luthe, W. (1961) Autogenic training, in Proceedings of the Third Congress of Psychiatry, Montreal.

Schutz, W. (1967) *Joy: Expanding Human Awareness.* Grove Press, New York.

Schwartz, G.E. (1971) Cardiac responses to self-induced thoughts. *Psychophysiology*, **8**, 462–7.

Schwartz, G.E. (1973) Pros and cons of meditation: anxiety, self control, drug abuse and creativity. Paper delivered at 81st Annual Convention of the American Psychological Association, Montreal.

Schwartz, G.E. (1975) Biofeedback, self-regulation and the patterning of physiological processes. *Am. Sci.*, **63**, 314–24.

Schwartz, G.E. and Goleman, D.J. (1976) Meditation as an alternative to drug use: accompanying personality changes. Unpublished paper, cited in Pelletier (1978).

Schwartz, G.E., Weinberger, D.A. and Singer, J.A. (1981) cardiovascular differentiation of happiness, sadness, anger and fear following imagery and exercise. *Psychosomatic Med.*, **43**, 343–64.

Schwarz, J. (1978) *Voluntary Controls: Exercises in Creative Meditation for the Activation of the Potential of the Chakras.* The Aletheia Foundation, New York.

Segalowitz, S.J. (1983) *Two Sides of the Brain.* Prentice Hall, Englewood Cliffs, New Jersey.

Selye, H. (1974) *Stress Without Distress.* Hodder & Stoughton, London.

Sergent, J. (1982) The cerebral balance of power: confrontation and cooperation. *J. Exp. Psychology: Human Perception Performance*, **8**, 253–72.

Serpell, J. (1990) Evidence of longterm effects of pet ownership on human health, in *Waltham Symposium 20: Pets, Benefits and Practice*, (ed. I.H. Burger), BVA Publications, Cambridge, pp. 2–4.

Serpell, J. (1991) Beneficial effects of pet ownership on some aspects of human health and behaviour. *J. R. Soc. Med.*, **84**, 717–20.

Shapiro, A.K. (1960) Contribution to a history of the placebo effect. *Behaviour Sci.*, **5**, 109–35.

Shapiro, A.K. and Morris, L.A. (1978) The placebo effect in medical and psychological therapies, in *Handbook of Psychotherapy and Behaviour Change*, (eds S.L. Garfield and A.E. Bergin), Wiley, New York.

Shaw, W.A. (1946) The relaxation of muscular action potentials to imaginal weightlifting. *Arch. Psychology*, **247**, 250.

Shea, J.D. (1985) Effects of absorption and instructions on heart rate control. *J. Mental Imagery*, **9**, 87–100.

Sheehan, P.W. (1972) *The Function and Nature of Imagery.* Academic Press, New York.

Sheikh, A.A. and Jordan, C.S. (1983) Clinical uses of mental imagery, in *Imagery: Current theory, Research and Application*, (ed. A.A. Sheikh), Wiley, New York, pp. 1–35.

Sheikh, A.A. (ed) (1984) *Imagination and Healing.* Baywood, Farmingdale, New York.

Sheikh, A.A., Kunzendorf, R.G. and Sheikh. K.S. (1989) Healing images: from ancient wisdom to modern science, in (eds A.A. Sheikh and K.S. Sheikh), *Eastern and Western Aproaches to Healing: Ancient Wisdom and Modern Knowledge*, Wiley, New York, pp. 470–515.

Sheikh, A.A. and Panagiotou, N.C. (1975) Use of mental imagery in psychotherapy: A critical review. *Perceptual Motor Skills*, **41**, 555–85.

Shekelle, R.B., Raynor, W.J., Ostfield, M.D. *et al.* (1981) Psychological depression and seventeen year risk of death from cancer. *Psychosomatic Med.*, **43**, 117–25.

Shepard, M. (1976) *Fritz: An Intimate Portrait of Fritz Perls and Gestalt Therapy.* Bantam, New York.

Shepard, R.N. (1975) Form, formation and transformation of internal representations, in *Information Processing and Cognition: The Loyola Symposium*, (ed. R. Solos), Erlbaum, Hillsdale, New Jersey.

Shepard, R.N. (1977) The mental image. *Am. Psychologist*, **33**, 125–37.

Shepard, R.N. and Chipman, S. (1970) Second-order isomorphism of internal representations: shapes of states. *Cognitive Psychology*, **1**, 1–17.

Shepard, R.N. and Cooper, L.A. (1975) Representation of colours in normal, blind and color blind subjects. Paper presented at Annual Meeting of the American Psychological Association Chicago 2 September, reported in Shepard (1977).

Shepard, R.N. and Cooper, L.A. (1982) *Mental Images and Their Transformations.* The MIT Press, Cambridge, Massachussetts.

Shepard, R.N. and Feng, F. (1972) A chronometric study of mental paper folding. *Cognitive Psychology*, 228–43.

Shepard, R.N. and Metzler, J. (1971) Mental rotation of three-dimensional objects. *Science*, **171**, 701–3.

Shepard, R.N., Kilpatrick, D.W. and Cunningham, J.P. (1975) The internal representation of numbers. *Cognitive Psychology*, **7**, 82–138.

Shorr, J.E. (1978) Clinical use of categories of therapeutic imagery, in *The Power of Human Imagination*, (eds J.S. Singer and K.S. Pope), Plenum, New York.

Shorr, J.E. (1983) *Psychotherapy Through Imagery.* Thieme-Stratton, New York.

Shotter, J. (1975) *Images of Man in Psychological Research.* Methuen, London.

Shuttleworth, E.C., Syring, V. and Allen, V. (1982) Further observations on the nature of prosopagnosia. *Brain Cognition*, **1**, 302–32.

Siebenthal, W. (1952) Eine vereinfachte Schwereubung des Schutz'schen autogenen trainings. *Ztschr. Psychother. Med. Psychol.*, **4** (2), 135.

Siegel, B.S. (1986) *Love, Medicine and Miracles.* Rider, London.

Siegel, B.S. (1990) *Peace, Love and Healing: Bodymind Communication and the Path to Self-healing.* Rider, London.

Silberman, E.K. and Weingartner, H. (1986) Hemispheric lateralization of functions related to emotion. *Brain Cognition*, **5**, 322–53.

Silverman, D. (1975) *Reading Castaneda: A Prologue to the Social Sciences.* Routledge and Kegan Paul, London.

Simonton, O.C. and Simonton, S.S. (1975) Belief systems and the management of the emotional aspects of malignancy. *J. Transpersonal Psychology*, **8**, 29–47.

Simonton, O.C., Matthews-Simonton, S. and Creighton. J. (1978) *Getting Well Again.* Bantam, New York.

Simonton, O.C. (1983) On the suffering of patients, families and caregivers. Presentation at Meet The Pioneers: understanding, preventing and controlling the effects of cancer. Conference of the Association for New Approaches to Cancer, London, 14 June.

Simonton, O.C., Matthews-Simonton, S. and Sparks, T.F. (1980) Psychological intervention in the treatment of cancer. *Psychosomatics*, **21**, 226–7.

Singer, J.L. (1974) Imagery and daydream methods, in *Psychotherapy and Behaviour Modification*, Academic Press, New York.

Singer, J.L. (1975) *Daydreaming and Fantasy*. George Allen and Unwin, London.

Singer, J.L. (1979) Imagery and affect in psychotherapy: elaborating private scripts and generating contexts, in *The Potential of Fantasy and Imagination*, (eds A.A. Sheikh and J.T. Shaffer), Brandon House, New York.

Smith, G.R. *et al.* (1985) Psychologic modulation of the human response to varicella zoster. *Arch. Int. Med.*, **145**, 2110–2.

Smith, D. and Over, R. (1987) Does fantasy-induced sexual behaviour habituate? *Behaviour Res. Therapy*, **25**, 477–85.

Snow, H.L. (1893) *Cancer and the Cancer Process*. Churchill, London.

Snyder, M. (1984) Progressive relaxation as a nursing intervention: an analysis. *Adv. Nursing Sci.*, **6** (3), 47–58.

Solomon, G.F. (1969) Emotions, stress, the CNS and immunity. *Ann. New York Acad. Sci.*, 335–42.

Somers, A.R. (1979) Mental status health – use of health services. *J. Am. Med. Assoc.*, **241**, 1818–22.

Spangler, D. (1977) *Revelation: the Birth of a New Age*. Findhorn Foundation, Scotland.

Spanos, N.P. (1982) A social psychological approach to hypnotic behaviour, in *Integrations of Clinical and Social Psychology*, (eds G. Weary and M.L. Mirels), Open University Press, Milton Keynes, pp. 227–31.

Spanos, N.P. (1986) Hypnosis and the modification of hypnotic sensibility: a social psychological perspective, in *What is Hypnosis? Current Theories and Research*, (ed. P.L.N. Naish), Open University Press, Milton Keynes, pp. 85–120.

Speigel, D. *et al.* (1989) Effect of psychosocial treatment on survival of patients with metastatic breast cancer. *Lancet*, 14 October, 888–91.

Sperry, R.W. (1962) Some general aspects of interhemispheric integration, in *Interhemispheric Relations and Cerebral Dominance Conference*, (ed. J. Young), Johns Hopkins University Press, Baltimore, Maryland.

Sperry, R.W. (1966) Hemispheric deconnection and unity in conscious awareness. *Am. Psychologist*, **23**, 723–33.

St. Exupéry, de, A. (1974) *The Little Prince*. Pan, London.

Stampfl, T.G. and Lewis, D.J. (1967) Essentials of Implosive Therapy: a learning theory based on psychodynamic behavioral therapy. *J. Abnormal Psychology*, **72**, 496–503.

Stern, J.A. *et al.* (1977) A comparison of hypnosis, acupuncture, morphin, valium, aspirin and placebo in the management of experimentally induced pain. *Ann. New York Acad. Sci.*, **296**, 175–93.

Stern, R.M. and Lewis, N.L. (1968) Ability of actors to control their GSRs and express emotions. *Psychophysiology*, **4**, 294–9.

Stevens, J.O. (1971) *Awareness: Exploring, Experimenting, Experiencing*. Real Peoples Press, Utah.

Stevens, J.O. (ed.) (1977) *Gestalt Is*. Bantam, New York.

Stock, W.E. and Geer, J.H. (1982) A study of fantasy-based sexual arousal in women. *Arch. Sexual Behaviour*, **11**, 33–47.

Stoll, B.A. (1979) Restraint of growth and spontaneous regression of cancer, in *Mind and Cancer Prognosis*, (ed. B.A. Stoll), Wiley, Chichester.

Storm, H. (1972) *Seven Arrows*. Ballantine, New York.

Storr, A. (1973) *Jung*. William Collins, Glasgow.

Storr, A. (1990) *Churchill's Black Dog: and Other Phenomena of the Human Mind*. Fontana, London.

Stovkis, B., Renes, B. and Landemann, H. (1961) Skin temperature under experimental stress and during Autogenic Training, in Proceedings of Third Conference of Psychiatry, Montreal.

Stoyva, J. (1976) Self-regulation: A context for biofeedback. *Biofeedback Self-regulation*, **1**, 1–6.

Stutley, M. (1985) *Hinduism: The Eternal Law: an Introduction to the Literature, Cosmology and Cults of the Hindu Religion*. Aquarian Press, Wellingborough, Northants.

Sugi, Y. and Akutsu, K. (1964) *Science of Zazen – Energy Metabolism*. Japan Publications, Tokyo.

Szasz, T.S. (1979) *The Myth of Psychotherapy: Mental Healing as Religion, Rhetoric and Repression*. Oxford University Press, Oxford.

Takahashi, H. (1984) Experimental study of self-control of heart rate: experiment for a biofeedback treatment of anxiety state. *J. Mental Health*, **31**, 109–25.

Tamez, E., Moore, M. and Brown, P. (1978) Relaxation training versus pro re nata medications. *Nursing Res.*, **27**, 160–4.

Tart, C.T. (1975) *Transpersonal Psychologies*. Routledge and Kegan Paul, London.

Taylor, A. (1987) *I Fly Out With Bright Feathers: The Quest of a Novice Healer*. Fontana/Collins, London.

Taylor, R. (1990) The immune system: guardian of our chemical identity. *Caduceus*, Winter, 26–30.

Temoshok, L. (1985) Biopsychosocial studies on cutaneous malignant melanoma: psychosocial factors associated with prognostic indicators, progression, psychophysiology and humor-host response. *Social Sci. Med.*, **20** (8), 833–40.

Temoshok, L. and Heller, B.W. (1981) Stress and 'Type C' versus epidemiological risk factors in melonoma. Paper presented at 89th Annual Convention of the American Psychological Association; Los Angeles, California, reported in Temoshok (1985).

Timms, M.W.H. (1989) Psychology and cancer: a historical review of pre-morbid factors with special reference to breast cancer. *Irish J. Psychology*, **10** (3), 411–25.

Trechmann, E.J. (translator) (1927) *The Essays of Montaigne*. Oxford University Press, London.

Tucker, D.M. *et al.* (1977) Right hemisphere activation during stress. *Neurophysiologia*, **15**, 697–700.

Van der Ploeg, H.M. (1988) Stressful medical events; a survey of patients' perceptions, in *Topics in Health Psychology*, (eds S. Maes, C.D. Spielberger, P.B. Defares and I.G. Sarons), Wiley, London, pp. 193–203.

Vaughan-Lee, L.(1992) The light hidden in the darkness: alchemical symbolism in dreams. *Caduceus*, **19**, 4–7.

Verbrugge, L.M. (1979) Marital status and health. *J. Marriage Family*, **41**, 267–85.

Vivekenanda, S. (1974) *Practical Vedanta*. Himalayas Advaita Ashrama, October.

Volicer, B.J. and Bohannon, M.W. (1975) A hospital stress rating scale. *Nursing Res.*, **24** (5), 352–9.

Von Franz, M.L. (1974) *Number and Time: Reflections Leading Towards a Unification of Psychology and Physics*. Rider, London.

Von Franz, M.L. (1975) *C.G. Jung. His Myth in Our Time.* Hodder & Stoughton, London.

Wagstaff, G.F. (1981) *Hypnosis, Compliance and Belief.* Harvester Press, Brighton.

Wagstaff, G.F. (1986) Hypnosis as compliance and belief: a socio-cognitive view, in *What is Hypnosis? Current Theories and Research,* (ed. P.L. Naish), Open University Press, Milton Keynes, pp. 59–84.

Wagstaff, G.F. (1987) Is hypnotherapy a placebo? *Br. J. Exp. Clin. Hypnosis,* **4** (3), 135–40.

Wallace, R.K. (1970) Physiological effects of transcendental Meditation. *Science,* **167,** 171–4.

Wallace, R.K. and Benson, H. (1972) The physiology of meditation, in *Altered States of Awareness: Readings from Scientific American,* W.H. Freeman, San francisco, pp. 125–31.

Warren, R.M. and Warren, R.P. (1969) *Helmhotz on Perception: its Physiology and Development.* Wiley, New York.

Waters, W.F. and McDonald, D.G. (1973) Autonomic response to auditory, visual and imagined stimuli in a systematic desensitization context. *Behaviour Res. Ther.,* **11,** 577–85.

Watson, J.B. (1916) The place of the conditioned reflex in psychology. *Psychological Review,* **23,** 89–116.

Watson, J.B. (1925) *Behaviourism.* Norton, New York.

Watson, L. (1973) *Supernature: the Natural History of the Supernatural.* Hodder & Stoughton, London.

Watson, L. (1976) *Gifts of Unknown Things.* Hodder & Stoughton, London.

Watts, A. (1961) *Psychotherapy East and West.* Pantheon, New York

Webb, J. (1980) *The Harmonious Circle: an Exploration of the Lives and Work of G.I. Gurdjieff, P.D. Ouspensky and Others.* Thames & Hudson, London.

Webster, C. (1988) The nineteenth century after-life of Paracelsus, in *Studies in the History of Alternative Medicine,* (ed. R. Cooper), MacMillan, London, pp. 79–88.

Wegner, N. and Zeaman, D. (1958) Strength of cardiac conditioned responses with varying unconditioned stimulus durations. *Psychological Review,* **65,** 238–41.

Wheatley, D. (1973) *The Devil and All His Works.* Beacon, Boston.

White, T., Holmes, D. and Bennett, D. (1977) Effects of instructions, biofeedback and cognitive activities on heart rate control. *J. Exp. Psychology: Human Learning Memory,* **3,** 477–84.

Wilber, K. (1984) *Quantum Questions.* Shambhala, Boulder, Colorado.

Wilhelm, R. (1978) *The I Ching or Book of Changes.* Routledge and Kegan Paul, London.

Willard, R.D. (1977) Breast enlargement through visual imagery and hypnosis. *Am. J. Clin. Hypnosis,* **19,** 195–200.

Williams, G.T. (1991) Programmed cell death: Apoptosis and oncogenesis. *Cell,* **65,** 1097–8.

Williams, J.M. *et al.* (1981) Sympathetic innervation of murine thymus and spleen: evidence for a functional link between the nervous and immune systems. *Brain Res. Bull.,* **6,** 83–94.

Wills, T.A. (1985) Supportive functions of interpersonal relations, in *Social Support and Health,* (eds S. Cohen and L. Syme), Academic Press, New York, pp. 61–78.

Windholz, M.J., Marmar, C.R. and Horowitz, M.J. (1985) A review of research on conjugal bereavement: impact on health and efficacy of intervention. *Comprehensive Psychiatry*, **26**, 433–47.

Wilson-Ross, N. (1973) *Hinduism, Buddhism, Zen*. Faber and Faber, London.

Wilson, V.S. (1987) Autogenic Training in the context of yoga, in *The Art of Survival: A Guide to Yoga Therapy*, (eds M.I. Gharote and M. Lockhart), Unwin Hyman, London, 116.

Wittstock, W. (1956) Untersuchungen uber cortikale Einflusse auf Korporienene Aktionstrome. *Psychiat. Neurol. Med. Psychol.*, **2/3**, 85.

Wolpe, J. (1969) *The Practice of Behaviour Therapy*. Pergamon, New York.

Wolpe, J. (1977) Systematic desensitization based on relaxation, in *Psychotherapies: a Comparative Casebook*, (eds S.J. Morse and R.I. Watson), Holt, Rinehart and Winston, New York, pp. 198–206.

Yaremko, R.M. and Butler, M.C. (1975) Imaginal experience and attenuation of the galvanic skin response to shock. *Bull. Psychonomic Soc.*, **5**, 317–8.

Zeltzer, L.K. (1980) The adolescent with cancer, in (ed. J. Kellerman), *Psychological Aspects of Childhood Cancer*, Chas C. Thomas, Springfield, Illinois.

Zukav, G. (1980) *The Dancing Wu-Li Masters: An Overview of the New Physics*. Fontana, London.

Index